SIGNS & STRATEGIES FOR EDUCATING STUDENTS WITH BRAIN INJURIES

A PRACTICAL GUIDE FOR TEACHERS AND PARENTS

Written by

Marilyn Lash, M.S.W., Gary Wolcott, M.Ed. & Sue Pearson, M.A.

LASH & ASSOCIATES PUBLISHING/TRAINING INC.

Item: SSES

Published by Lash & Associates Publishing/Training Inc.
100 Boardwalk Drive, Suite 150, Youngsville, NC 27596
Tel: (919) 556-0300

This book is part of a series on brain injury among children, adolescents, adults and veterans.
For a free catalog, contact Lash & Associates
Tel: (919) 556-0300 or visit our website *www.lapublishing.com*

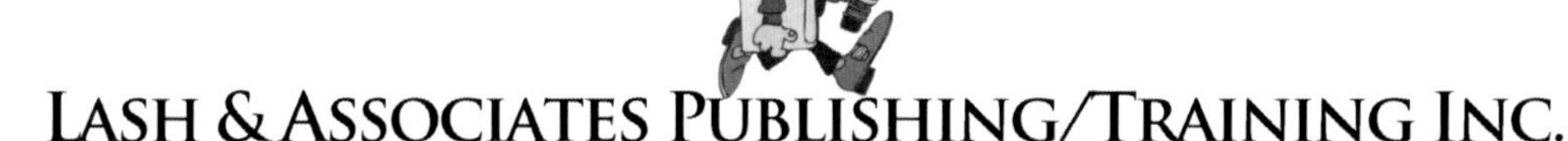

100 BOARDWALK DRIVE, SUITE 150, YOUNGSVILLE, NC 27596
TEL: (919) 556-0300 FAX: (919) 556-0900

WWW.LAPUBLISHING.COM

Table of Contents

Introduction

Finding the survivors of brain injury

In 1991, an amendment to the federal Individuals with Disabilities Education Act (IDEA) was passed. It created a category of traumatic brain injury to help educators identify these students and respond to their unique needs. The definition used under this law is

"...an acquired injury to the brain caused by an external physical force, resulting in total or partial functional disability or psychosocial impairment, or both, that adversely affects a child's educational performance. The term applies to open or closed head injuries resulting in impairments in one or more areas, such as cognition; language; memory; attention; reasoning; abstract thinking; judgment; problem-solving; sensory, perceptual, and motor abilities; psychosocial behavior; physical functions; information processing; and speech. The term does not apply to brain injuries that are congenital or degenerative, or to brain injuries induced by birth trauma." *(256B, 34CFR300)*

The National Center on Health Statistics reports that brain injury is the leading cause of disability in children between ages 1-14. Yet, in every state, the number of students receiving special education and related services with the classification of traumatic brain injury remains low in comparision to other conditions.

It has been estimated that up to 1,000,000 children receive brain injuries each year and that 1 in 500 children will be hospitalized with a brain injury each year. If the incidence of traumatic brain injury is so high, why is the number of students identified in the schools so low? Children who sustain mild brain injuries may not be identified at all, despite changes in their learning and behavior. Some students, whose injuries and resulting disabilities are more obvious, may be receiving services under other educational categories. Accurately identifying these students is a first and necessary step toward developing and providing the special education and support services they need in order to reach their potential for academic and vocational achievement, emotional growth, and preparation for adulthood. This book was written to help educators work through these critical issues.

Choice of words

The authors have several comments about terminology in this book. Although the federal law uses the term traumatic brain injury, there is another population of children with acquired brain injuries due to brain tumors, infections such as encephalitis and meningitis, and anoxic incidents such as near drownings, strangulation or suffocation. There are ongoing debates in many states about whether to use the limited traumatic definition of brain injury or to broaden this category to include all acquired brain injuries. While all states must comply with the federal definition, they have the option to use a broader definition under their state Department of Education's regulations.

The authors have chosen to use the term *brain injury* for this book. Our practical experience is that children with traumatic and acquired brain injuries share an interruption in the ongoing development of the brain. While the cause of the injury may differ, the consequences are similar in terms of the changes that parents and educators will see and in the child's ability to learn. Our use of the generic term brain injury includes both traumatic and acquired causes.

The other terms used often in this book are *family* and *parent*. They also are intended to be inclusive and recognize that the definition of family varies widely and includes many kinds of parents. The nuclear family with two parents is not the only model and is becoming less common. Single parents, step-parents, foster parents, adoptive parents, grandparents, and other relatives often are the primary caregivers who provide the emotional nurturing, physical care and supervision that all children need. Thus the term parent or family is intended to be inclusive and encompass all individuals who are closely involved in raising a child.

Finally, this book is a practical guide to help families and educators get started. Many checklists and worksheets have been designed so that you can apply the information to your child or your student. While the topic is complex, we have tried to present the information clearly with plenty of practical examples.

About the Authors

Marilyn Lash, M.S.W.

Currently a Director and founder of Lash and Associates Publishing/Training Inc., Marilyn is committed to providing practical information in user friendly language that is based on clinical research and best practices in the field. Her involvement of parents and educators in the development of this manual reflects a philosophy that families and schools must strive to work together to become partners in their role as service providers. Families and educators are pivotal partners in the student's development, recovery and education following a student's brain injury.

Marilyn's work over more than 30 years in medical, rehabilitation, educational and vocational settings has reinforced her belief that bridges need to be built between systems in order to avoid the fragmentation and frustration that families so commonly experience. Trained as a social worker at Boston University School of Social Work, she has experience as a clinician, researcher, trainer and administrator but her greatest interest is in program development.

She serves on various national and governmental task forces on brain injury and children with special needs to advise on health policy and research initiatives as well as on editorial boards of rehabilitation journals. Author of over 45 publications, Ms. Lash speaks nationally on psychosocial and educational issues for youths with brain injuries and their families.

Gary Wolcott, M.Ed.

An experienced counselor, administrator and trainer, Gary Wolcott has long been an advocate for families of children with brain injuries as well as a consultant with school systems. He was instrumental in raising the national awareness of rehabilitation professionals and educators about the long-term cognitive effects of brain injuries in children and their impact on learning.

He has been the Director of Education for the National Head Injury Foundation, founded a management and training consulting business, and worked as a researcher and educational specialist at the Research and Training Center in Rehabilitation and Childhood Trauma at Tufts-New England Medical Center in Boston.

Gary Wolcott is now based in the Portland, Maine area providing consultation and training services. He currently serves as Director of Education, Training and Staff Development at Goodwill Industries of Northern New England.

Sue Pearson, M.A.

Sue Pearson has worked as the state consultant for students with brain injuries for 12 years. Employed by the Iowa Department of Education, she worked with 15 brain injury resource teams across the state, creating communication networks with hospital and rehabilitation personnel, educational professionals and families. These networks continue to assist students with the transition from hospital based care to educational services in their local communities. The joint efforts of the Iowa Department of Education and the University of Iowa Center for Excellence on Disabilities serve as a model for other states to recognize and meet the special educational needs of students with brain injuries.

Trained as a special educator, Sue Pearson's major areas of study include orthopedic disabilities and learning disabilities. Building on her work in developmental disabilities for the past 25 years, she has conducted numerous workshop and conference presentations for educators, families and medical staff in Iowa and across the country. She has written extensively on the topic of school reentry and has been involved in the production of several training videos for educators and families, including Pieces of the Puzzle: An Introduction to Brain Injury.

Currently, Sue is employed by the University of Iowa as the Interdisciplinary Training Coordinator for the Iowa Leadership Education in Neurodevelopmental and Related Disabilities Program. This program is sponsored by the Maternal and Child Health Bureau and strives to train future leaders who will be working with children and young adults with disabilities.

Chapter 1
Helping Families

As children enter or return to school following a brain injury, parents expect that the worst is behind them. Few parents forget the horror of seeing their child injured and the fear that their child will not survive. Even years later, many parents can still describe in painful detail their feelings of anguish and helplessness during the agonizing wait for news at the hospital. Seeing their child lying unresponsive and comatose is a living nightmare for parents that is only magnified by feelings of guilt over failure to protect their child from harm.

Many parents spend long days and nights at the hospital while their other children manage as best they can at home, often in the substitute care of relatives or neighbors. More seriously injured children are often transferred from local hospitals to trauma centers in urban areas for specialized care. This creates even more upheaval in the family's life. Living in motel rooms, sleeping in hospital waiting rooms, and taking turns at their child's bedside are physically and emotionally exhausting. Many parents hang on simply by holding on to the hope that if they can only get their child home, then everything will be all right.

Families are unprepared for the physical, emotional, cognitive, and behavioral changes that can result from a brain injury. The grieving process that families experience is incomplete because the child survives but is changed. The process is further complicated by the many questions concerning prognosis that physicians and other health care professionals are unable to answer. Little research has been done to study the long-term outcomes of children after brain injuries.

This uncertainty creates many conflicts and anxieties for families. The tendency of many children to make remarkable physical progress often masks more subtle changes in the child's ability to process information, organize tasks, control impulses and monitor behaviors. For children whose brain injuries are considered less severe, and particularly those who did not have the dramatic stage of coma, subtle changes in emotions, behaviors and learning may puzzle families and educators. These difficulties usually become more apparent as the child enters or returns to school and is challenged to learn new information, adjust to multiple settings, interact with many students and teachers, and is expected to meet academic standards.

School is a critical environment for the child and family. It is the setting where children learn to function outside the shelter and protection of their homes and develop the social skills necessary for interpersonal relationships among peers. It is the arena where students gradually develop the skills and self-reliance that will enable them to become independent in preparation for adulthood. School also is the arena where the long-term and latent cognitive effects of a child's brain injury are most likely to become evident as the challenge of learning becomes increasingly complex.

The child with a brain injury is particularly at risk for lowered academic performance and social isolation which can then result in lowered self-esteem. Depression is a common reaction among students with brain injuries who are aware of their inability to achieve pre-injury levels of academic performance and social integration.

Educators are critical resources for interventions, guidance and support for students with brain injuries and for their parents and siblings. Educators can be the pivotal influence to prepare peers, develop support systems, identify needed interventions, design compensatory strategies, and develop academic and functional goals. It is important for educators to collaborate closely with parents or guardians throughout this process, yet too often the process of educational planning and negotiation for special education and related services becomes an adversarial one. Sometimes it begins too late and starts only after the student is failing. This chapter discusses primary concerns among families as their child returns to school and gives suggestions for how educators can help.

Blame and guilt

Motor vehicle collisions involving children as occupants or as pedestrians or bicyclists are a major cause of brain injuries. The force, speed and impact of these collisions directly contribute to the severity of the brain's injury. Falls from heights are another major cause of brain injuries among children. Common scenarios are falls down flights of stairs, out of windows, and off balconies. Again, the height from which the fall occurs is a factor in the severity of the injury.

Injuries are not isolated events. Not only may the child's brain be injured, but other body regions can be damaged as well. However, unlike bone fractures, cuts, bruises, and even internal injuries, brain injuries cause irreparable damage to the brain cells or neurons.

The physical damage to a child is compounded by the emotional aftermath. Other persons - parents, siblings or peers - may be injured and hospitalized as well. Just at the time when a young child may most need the comfort and presence of a parent, they may be separated for medical care. The death of a parent, sibling or peer can be devastating to the child who survives. The hospitalized child is even isolated from the mourning rituals of funerals. The full impact may not be felt until the child leaves the protective environment of the hospital and experiences the loss at home, in school and in the community.

The tragedy of these injuries is that they can be prevented. Children wearing safety belts, placed in child safety seats, and wearing bicycle helmets are less likely to be seriously injured. Safety measures such as protective rails and guards can protect children from falls. Parents experience terrible anguish and guilt over their failure to protect their child from harm as they relive "if only I had" thoughts.

A child's injury affects every member of the family in some way. The process of a family's grieving is unpredictable. Marital stress is common when spouses cope in different ways. Some parents recall feeling so totally overwhelmed that they isolated themselves at home, cried constantly and avoided friends and neighbors. Others coped by becoming "super busy" or becoming the supermom. As friends or teachers admired how well they were doing, they were terrified of falling apart if they stopped. In their grief, families may seek someone to blame who becomes the target of their anger. It is possible for schools or teachers to become this target just as a physician or nurse was at the hospital. It is important to understand that the anger stems from a deeper grief and rage about what has happened to the child.

Denial is a term used to describe the feeling that, *It can't be true, it's not real, it can't be as bad as they say*. Professionals in health care and educators often view denial as a negative symptom and become frustrated with parents because they "aren't facing the facts". Denial is actually a protective stage that helps families function as they gather the emotional strength to deal with their losses.

The word *acceptance* is often used, but does not reflect what a difficult and lengthy process it is for most families. How long it takes to reach this stage is different for each parent. One way of describing it is the point at which parents have an understanding of their child's abilities and limitations, of what they have lost and what is still unknown. It is that period when the injured child's condition and care are no longer the central focus in a family's life. While the child may always have special needs, they do not necessarily take priority over the needs of others in the family, but are balanced within the needs of all for care, attention, support and love.

How does rehabilitation differ for children?

Rehabilitation is a long-term process that continues throughout the child's development and has no defined end point. Discharge from a hospital or rehabilitation program does not signal a child's recovery. Rather, discharge from the hospital marks the beginning of the next stage of rehabilitation that occurs at home and in school.

Rehabilitation services are very different for children than for adults. There are still few pediatric rehabilitation programs specializing in brain injury. Those available may be far from the family's home. Many families are able to provide physical care at home despite the child's difficulties in mobility, dressing, bathing, speech, vision, hearing, cognition or behavior. Children are lighter and smaller; this enables families to provide care at home that would otherwise be impossible for adults.

Educators will encounter children with brain injuries who have spent many weeks or months in rehabilitation hospitals and programs before returning home. Many of these programs will contact the local school and involve them in the child's transition from hospital to home and return to school.

However, they will also meet children who return directly home from the acute care hospital or trauma center. *Length of stay in a hospital does not determine whether a child will need special education after a traumatic brain injury.* Similarly, the fact that a child was not treated in a rehabilitation program does not mean that the injury was not serious. The family whose child has returned directly home after a short hospital stay may be even *less* prepared to assess the long-term consequences of their child's injury and be *less* prepared to discuss educational needs with the school because they have not had the intervention of a rehabilitation team to communicate and work with the school.

Families lack prior experience with special education

The vast majority of children with brain injuries have no preexisting conditions. Consequently, their parents are inexperienced with the special needs system and many still consider it a program primarily for children with birth disorders or mental retardation.

The primary question that families ask is, "How will my child's brain injury affect his/her ability to learn?" Unfortunately, medical and rehabilitation experts can not give parents precise or definitive information. Although the Individuals with Disabilities Education Act (IDEA), specifically creates a special classification for children with traumatic brain injuries, the provision of services still needs to be negotiated individually with the child's local school.

Families need basic information about:

- What is special education?
- How do I apply for my child?
- How do I learn about my rights as a parent?
- What supports and services do my child need?
- How can I get to know and develop a sense of confidence in the educational team?
- How can I tell if my child is learning?
- How can I measure my child's progress?

Concerns about qualifications of educators

Families often refer to discharge from the hospital or rehabilitation program as the second crisis of injury because the responsibility for the child's ongoing care and continuing needs shifts to them. During the medical crisis, families draw reassurance from the multiple specialists caring for their child. Knowing that their child is in the hands of experts brings some comfort. By contrast, when the child returns to school, families typically find that educators and school staff have little or no prior experience or training in brain injury. This creates considerable anxiety and even alarm. "How will the school know what my child needs if they've never had a student with a brain injury before?"

The time required by schools to gather medical information, complete testing, determine eligibility, and construct educational plans often takes much longer than families expect. It contrasts with the rapid pace of the child's earlier medical treatment. Meanwhile, many parents become anxious about the effects of these delays upon their child's academic progress and emotional adjustment.

Educators can build confidence in parents by showing an interest and willingness to learn about the effects of brain injuries. Parents stress that the interest, flexibility and commitment of teachers can foster positive relationships. While parents may prefer that teachers already have specialized skills and training in brain injuries, many recognize that teachers can acquire this knowledge. When teachers are receptive to suggestions for reading, obtain information from state brain injury associations, make themselves available for consultation with experts, inquire about strategies used by parents, and ask insightful questions, then many parents are reassured and feel that their child is less "at risk" in school.

Timing of child's return to school

The length of a child's hospitalization is not a predictor of what the child will need upon returning to school. The severity of the initial injury is not the same as the severity of the resulting disability. Some very seriously injured children recover quite well. Others with less severe brain injuries have long lasting difficulties. The length of time that a child is absent following an injury, however, can affect how educators and families perceive the child's needs. When a child is in critical condition, particularly when a coma extends for weeks or months, schools are alerted to the possibility that this child may have a serious disability. The child who is seen briefly in the emergency department and sent home, or admitted overnight for observation, is more readily assumed to be "all right." This is not always true.

Each brain injury is different. Any child whose behaviors and performance at school change following a blow to the head needs to be evaluated for a traumatic brain injury.

The transfer of information between medical specialists and educators frequently is problematic. School staff often assume that medical staff will advise them of what is needed, while medical staff may assume that the school will know what to do. Too often, the result is poor communication and planning between hospitals and schools. When schools do receive medical reports, they are frequently written in such technical medical jargon that they are of little use for educational planning. This widens the gap in communication.

Medical and educational institutions are completely different entities in terms of how they are staffed, financed and operated. These fundamental differences can lead to conflicts in expectations and goals as the injured child moves from one setting to the other. Thus, families become the link for information between hospital staff, follow-up appointments and school staff. However, families may not know what information is needed, how to collect it, and what to do with it. This new responsibility is now added to the many changes and stresses already affecting the family.

Miracle of survival

Families frequently describe their child's survival and recovery from a life threatening injury as miraculous. Having seen their child close to death - in a coma - on a respirator - wired to machines and attached to tubes everywhere, is a terrifying experience. Even when their child slowly emerged from coma, many families were given cautious predictions about their functional abilities for mobility, speech, communication and self-care. Having watched a child beat the grim odds given by medical experts, it is not surprising that many parents expect the same miraculous recovery to extend into school.

This need to hope is also a reflection of how weary and exhausted families can be by the time a child is ready to return to school. Going to school may signal a respite for families from the child's daily care and supervision, and from the stress of lowered finances due to time off from work and unpaid medical bills. Consequently, many families are unprepared to face the difficulties that their child now has in school. If the school adopts an attitude of "Let's wait and see" how the child does in school, the family may be only too willing to "hope for the best" because they are exhausted. However, this delay can result in lost opportunities for early intervention for educational planning and the student may be quickly discouraged by early failures and difficulties adjusting to the demands of the classroom and curriculum.

Families need careful and supportive guidance by school staff to make sure that the child's needs are thoroughly assessed and that educational plans are designed as soon as possible to address the child's special learning needs. The initial "honeymoon period" between educators and families often bursts when it becomes evident that the child is having serious difficulties and parents feel that the school is too slow to react. Too often, negotiations deteriorate into legal battles between schools and families. The following suggestions are designed to prevent this from occurring and to encourage a partnership for educational planning between parents and educators.

Action steps for educators

Listen to families

Parents know their child best. They not only have the pre-injury comparison of how their child is functioning, but they have seen their child's reactions and progress through the various stages of treatment and recovery. Parents can detect subtle changes before they are apparent to others. This is particularly important with younger children who are unable to express their needs clearly. Families also have opportunities to observe their child's cognitive progress in many different settings and circumstances. They see how their child functions during days and evenings, when tired or alert, in concentrated silence or with distracting interruptions. Parents and family members have experience in developing cueing systems, designing strategies to aid memory, and helping children finish tasks. Parents' observations may yield information that is far more practical than testing and achievement scores that represent the child's capacity in a structured and controlled setting.

Carry over and consistency between families and educators are essential for the child with a brain injury. Therefore, it is important for educators and families to share their methods so that the family can reinforce effective techniques used in the classroom. Similarly, educators may find home based strategies that parents have found effective when modified to the classroom.

Help parents set up a record keeping system

A child's recovery is likely to extend over years. Families will meet with many specialists, educators, and consultants. Children will have many assessments done, testing performed, reports written and recommendations made. None of this information is likely to be stored in one place and can be just about impossible to track down years later. As students progress through grades and various schools, bits and pieces inevitably get lost or separated. Parents and family members will be the only constant source of historical information over the years that can influence the student's access to services and support.

Families and educators can benefit right in the beginning by setting up an educational record in a flexible three ring binder that remains the property of the parent. This record will grow as the child moves from teacher to teacher, grade to grade and school to school. Educators and families can strategize what information is most useful to record. This can provide a critical and comprehensive record that can be used by families and educators to track a child's progress, compare interventions and program results, and record important dates, names and addresses. It provides a continuous record that can be useful to identify patterns, spot potential problems and compare programs and results.

Suggestions for sections to include are:

- ☐ description of pre-injury abilities and performance in school and at home
- ☐ description of medical care and rehabilitation
- ☐ reports by consultants and specialists
- ☐ description of current medications and record of past medications (note any special problems)
- ☐ community resources
- ☐ state and federal programs
- ☐ description of current strengths and needs
- ☐ past and current academic grades and performance

- ☐ special education directors, teachers, teacher aids, and tutors
- ☐ special education services recommended and received
- ☐ related services such as transportation, therapies, counseling, etc.
- ☐ special interests and hobbies of the student
- ☐ successful interventions

Tip - Date each entry for an accurate record over time.

Provide support as students and parents alter hopes and dreams

Uncertainty about the future is one of the most difficult aspects of brain injury for families. The loss of hopes and dreams is painful. The age when the child is injured is a factor. Parents of children who were injured when very young talk about lost potential. When preschool age children are injured, or even very young elementary school children, so much is still unknown about the child's skills, abilities and interests. The child's personality is still emerging as communication skills develop, habits form, and unique character traits appear. Parents speak wistfully of not knowing how their child "might have been" had the injury not occurred.

A particular sadness expressed by parents of children with severe disabilities caused by injuries during their formative years is the sadness of watching younger siblings surpass them. Siblings of children injured at a young age also quickly lose their recall of the child prior to injury.

Parents also talk about recurring depression or sadness as their child approaches developmental milestones such as starting kindergarten, learning to read or ride a bike, dating, and graduation.

Aspirations for jobs, vocational training, careers, and college already may be defined for the older child, especially for adolescents. A brain injury may seriously threaten these plans and force families, students and educators to reevaluate them. Peer pressure among adolescents can make it especially difficult for the student with a brain injury to fit in and keep up with classmates. Appearance, dating, and sexuality become primary concerns among adolescents. The student with a brain injury may no longer be as attractive to and accepted by peers.

Too many high school students injured close to graduation accept high school diplomas without realizing that this disqualifies them for additional special educational services. This premature graduation can readily backfire as students find that vocational rehabilitation services in the community are not as readily available as special education in public schools. Any family with an adolescent approaching graduation age needs careful advice and guidance from educators to insure that transition plans and programs effectively prepare the student for adulthood.

Recognize limits of information among foster families

Child abuse is a primary cause of brain injury among infants and preschool children. Foster and adoptive families typically lack complete medical records and family histories for these children. Many children who have been physically abused have multiple disabilities including damaged vision or hearing as well as motor and cognitive difficulties. Multiple foster homes and temporary placements can contribute to behavioral problems and exacerbate emotional disturbances among these children. This can contribute to delinquent patterns and even expulsion from school. Because children's brains are especially vulnerable to injury if abuse occurs at an early age, it is important for foster families and educators to question the relationship between early physical abuse and later learning and behavioral difficulties.

Remember siblings and encourage parents to evaluate their needs

Brothers and sisters are often the forgotten victims. With the primary concern and attention directed at the injured child, siblings easily can be overlooked. The turmoil at home inevitably affects siblings. Young siblings mistakenly may believe they are responsible for the injury since young children's magical thinking often confuses cause and effect. Siblings may have witnessed the injury and have recurrent nightmares, fears, or trouble sleeping. Siblings may be jealous of the attention focused on the injured child and angry at disruptions in the family's routine. They may also feel embarressed about changes in their siblings's behavior, particularly in public places. Older siblings may have additional responsibilities of caring for others and managing the household while parents are at the hospital.

These stresses may become evident at school as the grades of siblings drop, as attention wanders, or as behaviors change. Families may fail to inform the teachers of siblings about the family crisis. Consequently, it is important to inform the teachers of siblings when schools are advised of a child's injury. School staff can then be alert to changes in siblings' behavior and grades and provide additional attention, support, and counseling.

A final comment

Families and educators share the goal of helping the student learn, develop skills, and explore potential. This can best be done as partners in planning, educating, and evaluating the student's needs, abilities and difficulties. When a student has special educational needs as a result of a brain injury, this partnership between families and educators becomes even more important. Each has an expertise and viewpoint that can help guide the student, develop effective plans, and bring insight to work through difficulties and find needed resources. After all, both parents and educators share the ultimate goal of preparing the student for adulthood.

Chapter 2
Sorting Out Myths and Facts

Parents and teachers often are unfamiliar with the immediate and long-term effects of brain injuries upon students. The needs and responses of these students are sometimes very different than those of children and youth with other disabilities. Developments in medical care, rehabilitation, and educational services within the last decade have made it possible for most children and adolescents with moderate and severe disabilities due to brain injuries to return home and go to school. Likewise, many individuals with mild brain injuries, who were once assumed to be "okay", are now known to be at risk for educational and behavioral difficulties. It is vital that the unique changes resulting from brain injuries be understood by each person in the student's world. The following misunderstandings often create barriers to effective educational and supportive services for students.

MYTH: ***All brain injuries are the same.***

FACT: No two brain injuries are alike. A brain injury is not like any other injury or disease. The brain is very complex and recovery from an injury depends on what areas of the brain were damaged and how severely. Damage can be caused by swelling and bruising of the brain, blood clots, shearing and tearing of nerve fibers, infection, reduction in the supply of oxygen, and death of brain cells.

WHAT TO DO: Ask parents to provide copies of written information such as hospital discharge summaries or reports by specialists such as neurologists, neuropsychologists, physical therapists, occupational therapists, speech and language pathologists or other specialists. Ask parents to describe how they think the injury has affected their child and to describe what changes they see at home and in school.

> *Joan sustained a brain injury while riding her bike and I'm not sure what to do or how to help her. She's not like the student I had last year in my home room. Although both students were hurt while riding their bikes, that's about all they have in common. It feels like I'm learning about the effects of brain injury all over again.*

MYTH: ***Physical recovery is a sign that the brain has healed.***

FACT: The student with a brain injury may show no outward signs of disability. Difficulties with short-term memory, focusing attention, or following directions are not as readily obvious as physical changes in walking or loss of speech. While broken bones and cuts heal with the growth of new skin and bone, the brain does not produce new neurons or brain cells. Many children have dramatic physical recoveries that parents often describe as miraculous, but cognitive recovery is a much slower process. The appearance of well-being is deceptive. As a result, the brain injury may not be recognized by educators or the student may be described as lazy or unmotivated. Special learning needs may go unrecognized and contribute to the student's later frustration and failure.

WHAT TO DO: Carefully observe the student's social behavior, classroom performance and ability to do age appropriate tasks. Educators, psychologists, and rehabilitation therapists, who have training and experience evaluating children and adolescents with brain injuries, can identify injury-related problems in learning and behavior. Parents can help by describing changes in their child since the injury. Develop an individualized educational plan based on the unique strengths and needs of the student.

Steve had a brain injury at age 6 when he was struck by a car while playing on the sidewalk. Initially, he couldn't recall the names for many common objects and didn't recognize his parents or sisters. Within a few weeks, however, these abilities improved and his physical recovery was quite good.

His teacher and parents were surprised when he began having difficulty with what seemed to be simple tasks at home and in school. Once an easygoing child, he now had frequent temper outbursts and sometimes became physically aggressive. His reading skills were relatively good, but his comprehension was poor, which resulted in problems with his written work. The changes in Steve's behavior were attributed to his overdependence on others for help during his long hospital stay. A behavior management program was developed, but failed to make any improvements.

Although Steve's physical recovery was excellent, his cognitive recovery lagged far behind. Impairment of his memory made it hard to learn at school and to remember instructions and directions at home. When this was interpreted as misbehavior, he was frustrated. Once Steve's problems were accurately identified, adaptations for reading comprehension were made and a buddy system was put in place at school. By adjusting expectations at home and school, Steve was more successful.

MYTH: ***The student with a severe brain injury will be seriously disabled.***

FACT: Length of coma and post traumatic amnesia are two indicators of an injury's severity. The severity of the student's brain injury, however, does not necessarily predict what the long term outcome will be. When the period of coma lasts for more than 24 hours, this is an indicator that the brain injury is severe and increases the likelihood of long-term difficulties in behavior, learning, emotional well-being, social skills and physical abilities. Although it is estimated that only 10 to 20% of brain injuries are classified as severe, within that group up to 80% are likely to have multiple long-term impairments. Patterns of recovery vary and much depends on what areas of the brain are damaged. There are no precise predictors of outcomes. There is a common stereotype that a person with a severe brain injury will be severely physically disabled. In fact, children tend to make rapid physical progress but long-term difficulties in behavior and learning are much more common.

WHAT TO DO: Learn as much as you can from parents, hospital and rehabilitation experts about the student's injuries and recovery. Information about the student's pre-injury performance can help identify current strengths and new needs. When possible, speak directly with the medical and rehabilitation team that cared for the student. Gather enough information and records to develop a complete picture of the student's needs and strengths. Base the student's educational program on identified strengths and needs, not on the severity of the initial injury.

Regardless of how long it has been since the injury, always inquire about its severity and the length of coma. No matter how "good" the student looks, a severe brain injury is an indicator that there are likely to be cognitive changes that will affect learning.

A motor vehicle crash involving two cars left Mary Ann with a severe brain injury. After she emerged from coma, her memory was impaired and she became frustrated when she was unable to recall the names for everyday objects. Her social skills were frequently inappropriate and she made offensive comments to friends. Previously a talented pianist, she now found it hard to play simple tunes. Like many, Mary Ann showed great improvement during the first two years after her accident. However, her circle of friends decreased and she spend a lot of time by herself. She continued to have difficulty with academic work and abandoned her music altogether.

Several years later, Mary Ann and her parents continue to notice small improvements in many areas. They feel, as do her teachers, that a structured social skills group and a few special friends have helped her relearn some critical skills and her social life is slowly improving. They have also seen her interest in the piano return and gradually she has been able to read more difficult music. Although her rate of progress is not as rapid as it was initially, there has been steady improvement in many areas.

MYTH: ***The student with a mild traumatic brain injury will have no problems recovering.***

FACT: The terms mild brain injury and concussion are often used interchangeably. With both, there is no loss of consciousness or it is lost very briefly for seconds or minutes. Concussions are common with falls and sports injuries. The youth may seem stunned, dazed or briefly confused

Many children with concussions are examined in Emergency Departments or the doctor's office and have normal findings on neurological examinations. For many years, it was thought that no damage to the brain occurred and there were no long-term consequences. Recent research shows that even these so called "mild" brain injuries can have serious effects on thinking, memory, and behavior.

A student with a mild brain injury may have subtle problems that go unrecognized, especially if the student was not hospitalized. The student, parents and teachers may notice unexplained difficulties. Headaches, difficulty concentrating, mood swings, a "feeling of not being myself," may be indicators of a brain injury that needs to be evaluated by a specialist with experience in mild traumatic brain injuries. While most symptoms resolve in 6 to 8 weeks, some students have long-term difficulties and require special services in school.

WHAT TO DO: Take any signs of change seriously. Encourage the student and parents to see a physician familiar with the effects of concussion. A neuropsychological evaluation may also help define subtle learning and thinking problems and identify educational and behavioral strategies to help the student.

Jeff fell out of a tree house when he was 8 years old and his brain injury went undiagnosed for almost a year. Although he didn't lose consciousness, medical reports describe him as being unresponsive right after the fall and disoriented for a few days afterward. It seemed his only serious injury was a broken arm and a few bruised ribs, and he returned to school 10 days later.

Right away, he began having academic and behavior problems. He failed at things that previously had been easy and was unable to concentrate. His mother was worried about his frequent headaches and what she thought might be depression although she didn't understand why he would be depressed. Jeff admitted that he often felt like crying but couldn't explain why.

A year after his fall, a neurologist found that his brain injury was more significant than initially thought. Medication was prescribed for his depression and attention problems and he got some extra help at school with an aide.

MYTH: ***Younger students recover better from their injuries.***

FACT: The brain is still developing right up through adolescence. Younger children are at greater risk for difficulties in the future because the ongoing development of the brain has been interrupted. The younger the child, the more immature and vulnerable the brain is to an injury.

The brain's ability to "rewire" itself is not well understood. While previously learned skills are often left largely intact after a brain injury, acquiring new skills is a common problem. When a child is injured at a young age, fewer basic living and educational skills have been acquired than in an older child or young adult. Lacking this foundation, the young child cannot draw on previously mastered skills to compensate for changes caused by an injury.

It takes longer to see the effects of a brain injury in a young child because basic skills like language, arithmetic, reading and writing are still being learned. Reliance on adults for supervision and guidance protects the younger child and helps this child compensate. However, as this child grows up and is expected to become more independent and responsible, difficulties with problem solving, planning and organizing often become apparent.

Different lobes of the brain develop at different times as the child matures. As this development occurs, the effects of earlier damage from an injury become apparent. Thus, it takes longer for the effects of the brain injury to appear in children. Unlike the familiar saying, "Time heals all wounds," time *reveals* the effects of a brain injury in childhood.

WHAT TO DO: Early intervention is vital for a younger student with a brain injury. Regular evaluation by developmental specialists who are experienced in brain injury can help identify problems that might be overlooked in a preschool setting. An early intervention program can help the student build critical skills for later school years.

As time passes, the link between an earlier brain injury and new difficulties is often lost. Whenever there are changes in skills and abilities or new difficulties with learning or behavior, a neuropsychological assessment can help determine the relationship between the earlier injury and current difficulties and needs.

When you meet with parents, ask questions that may provide information about a previous brain injury. Sometimes finding out how a student was hurt may indicate that an earlier brain injury has been overlooked.

Possible questions include, Has your child ever been in a car crash? Had a serious fall? Been dazed or confused after a sports accident, or lost consciousness? If so, encourage parents to follow up with a physician experienced in brain injury.

Mary fell off a tractor while visiting her uncle's farm when she was 3. Her brain injury was severe and resulted in cognitive impairments and paralysis of her left side. Because she was hurt before she learned how to care for herself, her acquired cognitive and physical impairments made feeding and dressing even harder for her. She also had no prior experience with reading and math and found academic activities challenging.

She was fortunate to attend a preschool for children with special needs and the teacher identified many helpful strategies and adaptations. This information was communicated to her kindergarten teacher who had assumed her condition was birth related until she learned about her brain injury. The strategies identified for her were helpful for easing Mary's transition into the more formal classroom setting.

MYTH: ***After seven or eight months, a student with a brain injury will not improve anymore because the brain's repair mechanisms have shut down.***

FACT: There is no timetable for recovery. Rapid changes occur most often in the first 6 months after an injury and continue at a slower rate throughout the first year. Reaching a plateau does not mean the end of progress. It means that the child is moving into the next stage of long-term recovery that will be more gradual. Progress can continue for months and years. It may be slower and new difficulties may appear as the student attempts more complex tasks, but progress can continue indefinitely.

WHAT TO DO: Predictions based on arbitrary time frames can create barriers for the student and discourage educators and families. Focus on the student's current abilities and what assistance is needed in the short term. Build the student's educational plan upon the functional performance within the school environment and ongoing information acquired from assessment by educational and allied health professionals.

Doctors did not expect Michelle to live after prolonged swelling caused severe damage to her brain. Everyone, including her parents, was surprised when her medical condition stabilized and she began the slow process of recovery. Her parents were told that Michelle would probably not be able to walk or talk and would most likely have "no real quality of life".

Within a few months, Michelle was walking and talking and returned to school. She attended regular classes, received specialized assistance from an instructional aide, but made little progress in academic work after several months of instruction.

The teacher felt that Michelle's parents were in denial when they insisted that she be maintained in the regular classroom and that she receive extended year programming.

They hired a tutor for the summer and after about 6 months, Michelle began to make steady progress in reading. Not only did she begin to maintain a sight word vocabulary, but she looked for books at the library. Her most significant progress in reading occurred almost two years after her injury.

MYTH: ***A brain injury erases your memory.***

FACT: Usually a student with a brain injury will retain most previous learning and knowledge. Difficulty learning new information is a more common problem. A student may have posttraumatic amnesia which is the inability to recall events just before and after the injury. A student may have gaps in memory and skills and appear confused at times. Skills may seem contradictory with great strengths in some areas and major difficulties in others.

WHAT TO DO: Work with the student to identify which concepts and skills are intact. Use this information to enhance the student's educational program by building on these strengths.

Some of the student's peers may expect that their friend will not remember anything upon coming home from the hospital and returning to school. Others may be surprised at the changes they observe. Talk with the student's peers about their expectations and fears. Discuss ways in which they can support their friend.

Jamie was injured in a summer bicycle collision when he hit a pothole and ran into a tree. Although he had a moderate brain injury, he recovered rather quickly. In September, he returned to school and seemed to be doing relatively well, both social and academically. As the semester continued, however, his teachers noticed that he was having more difficulty with assignments.

On investigation, it appeared that Jamie's initial academic success may have occurred during the first few weeks of school because the time was spent reviewing material that had been presented the year before. Like many individuals, Jamie was more successful in relearning previously learned information.

Once the students began working on new concepts and skills, he was less successful. Although he was able to make progress with new material, teachers found that his learning rate was slower than it had been in the past, which was frustrating for him. By modifying some of his assignments and providing additional organization and structure, he was more successful.

MYTH: ***Denial of the disability or problem is bad. The student and family must face the harsh reality of a disability in order to adjust.***

FACT: Denial comes in many forms for many different reasons. A student's brain injury may affect self-awareness. The injury may limit the student's understanding and insight. On the other hand, denial may be an emotional self-defense that is needed by the student.

Denial is an expected and normal coping response among survivors and families. Parents are often labeled as being in denial when they refuse to acknowledge their child's difficulties or have what others view as unrealistic expectations for recovery. Professionals sometimes misinterpret parents' intense hopes and beliefs as a denial of the disability. Parents and students often need to hold onto this hope as they gather their strength to face the unknown future.

WHAT TO DO: Give the family time to adjust to all the changes that have occurred. Some families adjust more quickly than others. Use the goals identified by the student or parents. Then break the goals down into small practical, educational steps. This allows the family and student to use time and their experience to build a more realistic view of the student's abilities and needs. Denial of a disability may be damaging if parents (or children) develop unrealistic expectations that lead to repeated failure. However all of us have ideas and dreams about what we want to be able to do and all of us have, at some point, been allowed to try and fail. It is a natural part of life and the learning process.

Justin's parents felt he was being unrealistic when he decided to return to college after his brain injury. They recognized personality changes and memory problems and were concerned about his ability to manage his academic work and personal life. After months of family arguments, they agreed to let him try.

Justin returned to school the following semester, intent on carrying a full academic load. After the first quarter, he realized he couldn't keep up and decided to drop three classes. This helped him do reasonably well although he admitted that his grades were still not as good as before and he was working much harder just to keep up. Justin's parents now feel that it was a good idea to let him return to college. Although they recognize that his abilities are different now, they feel he is making good progress and see that his self-esteem has improved.

MYTH: ***Normal IQ scores after a brain injury mean that the child will have no problems learning in school.***

FACT: IQ scores are not accurate predictors of learning after a brain injury. Intelligence tests that produce IQ scores have long been used in schools to evaluate students. Students with brain injuries often have test scores within what is considered the "normal" range of intelligence.

This is misleading because many intelligence tests focus on recalling old information that is stored in the brain. Many children with brain injuries do quite well on these tests. However, it is the ability to learn *new* information that often changes after a brain injury. This is less likely to show up on standard intelligence tests.

A child with a brain injury is also likely to do better in the quiet testing room with one-to-one instruction by the examiner. This same child may not do as well in the classroom when attention, planning and organization are easily interrupted by noise and distractions.

WHAT TO DO: Arrange to have a neuropsychological evaluation completed which will examine the relationships between the brain and behavior and gives a more accurate analysis of the child's ability to learn and function in school.

As a result of the standardized testing done at school, Adam's teachers concluded that his academic problems were the result of poor motivation, since he scored well above average and had previously received good grades.

Neuropsychological testing revealed that Adam's earlier injury was affecting his abilities in spatial relationships, abstract reasoning and problem-solving. His success in earlier grades drew on his strengths with lots of memorization and repetition. The nature of the work in junior high school required more complex analytical thought and abstract reasoning, processes that showed significant impairment during testing. His high marks on intelligence testing reflected his strengths and information in stored memory. When the neuropsychologist conducted more specific tests designed to identify how well the damaged parts of his brain were functioning, a different profile emerged.

MYTH: ***Professionals are always the final experts.***

FACT: Parents know their child best. Only parents have had first hand experience with their child before and after the brain injury. They have seen their child through every stage of care and have watched their child progress over time. Professionals come and go. Programs change. Parents are the only constant in the child's life. Involve parents in the educational process and work with them as partners rather than adversaries.

WHAT TO DO: Help parents understand the process of special education and their roles and rights under the law by providing them with the state's handbook or manual written for parents. Introduce them to other parents or programs that provide information and support. For many parents, special education is an entirely new system that can seem confusing, frustrating and overwhelming.

Involve parents as early as possible by asking them to share their experience, perspective and knowledge of their child. Ask them to describe how they believe their child has changed since the brain injury and what their hopes are for the future. Most parents have worked out methods at home to help their child compensate and adapt. Find out what these are and talk with parents about how they might be used in the classroom. Many parents have done extensive reading about brain injury and found resources in the community. Ask them to share this information with you. You can help parents learn about special education and they can help you learn about brain injury.

The teachers who had the greatest impact were the ones who admitted what they didn't know but took a special interest in our child and were willing to learn about brain injury. At first, we were nervous because the school seemed so inexperienced, but we didn't know anything either before Sam got hurt. The other thing that makes a difference is when teachers recognize that we have information to contribute and include us in the process. I get tired of being a squeaky wheel with some of them, but I'll do it when I have to. It's so much easier when we can work together from the beginning and that's when Sam really benefits.

A Parent

Chapter 3
Signs and Changes to Watch for in Students with Brain Injuries

This section helps school staff, especially teachers, prepare and problem solve as they identify, teach and coordinate educational programs for students with brain injuries. Teachers are the experts in education but they may have little training or knowledge about brain injury. By contrast, medical and rehabilitation professionals may have special expertise in brain injury, but are often unfamiliar with the system known as special education. The information presented here helps bridge the gap between rehabilitation programs and schools. Its goal is to help teachers understand how a brain injury can affect a student's abilities and performance at school.

Much is still unknown about the long-term effects of brain injuries to children. We are just beginning to study and understand how an injury can alter the brain's development over time and affect the student's ability to learn. Many of these children, especially those with moderate to severe brain injuries, did not survive 15-20 years ago. The development of pediatric trauma centers and advances in trauma medicine, neurosurgery, and emergency medical services have changed this.

A student's recovery from a brain injury is hard to predict. Each injury is so different and much depends on the areas of the brain that are affected. The level of academic and social functioning of the child before the injury can be a significant factor. The age of the student when injured is also a factor since a child's brain continues to develop and organize through adolescence. When injuries interrupt normal developmental patterns and milestones, it can affect subsequent stages of development. Some difficulties do not appear for months or years after an injury. As the brain matures, the effects of an earlier injury become apparent in school.

Changes to watch for when a student has a brain injury

The educational plan should be a flexible guide that reflects changes as students progress and recover from brain injuries. Goals, abilities, and difficulties change for all children as they grow. Learning is a continual process that is never complete for any individual. For children with brain injuries, this process is more complex. The injury can have different effects at various times during the student's education. As the student advances through grades, the complexity of learning increases and different abilities and skills are required.

It is most important that parents, educators and rehabilitation specialists work as a team with these students. Teachers are in critical positions to influence the student's opportunities for success in school. Depending on the school and classroom, the teacher may be with the student from one to six hours a day. This gives the teacher a unique opportunity to assess the student's abilities as well as difficulties. It also places a major responsibility on the teacher to figure out how the brain injury has affected the student and to determine how to help this student learn. This is not an easy challenge.

Families who are accustomed to the intensive and individualized care that their child received in the hospital and rehabilitation setting are often concerned about how their child will do in the classroom where there are more students and less individual attention. Teachers must address the needs of many students in the classroom, including those who require specialized assistance, and it is a constant challenge to meet the variety of student needs.

Less intensive therapy services in schools are frequently misinterpreted by families as inadequate. In fact, they are usually an indication of the student's progress to a later stage of recovery where less intensive services are needed. But this shift also reflects the student's transition from physical, occupational and speech therapies that are designed for medical rehabilitation to therapies provided in the school setting that are related to educational needs. This distinction is often confusing for parents, and needs clarification by the educational team when the child returns to school.

Many of the emotions, behaviors and reactions that students experience after a brain injury can cause problems at school if they are not recognized or are misunderstood. The most common changes are described in this chapter with suggestions to help teachers identify them. This is the first step toward developing effective teaching and learning strategies.

Changes often seen in students with a brain injury include:

- ☐ cognitive and physical fatigue
- ☐ irritability and anger
- ☐ passive behavior
- ☐ depression
- ☐ social immaturity
- ☐ sexual inappropriateness
- ☐ forgetfulness
- ☐ easily distracted
- ☐ poor organization

Cognitive and physical fatigue

This is a very common long-term effect, and is often most pronounced during the early stages of recovery when the student first returns to school. Fatigue is more than a physical effect. It can also affect cognitive functions, emotional stability and physical skills. Any difficulties in these areas will become more noticeable when the student is tired. For example, a student with one-sided weakness may be more likely to stumble when tired or handwriting may be harder to read. Reading comprehension may be more difficult or speech slower.

Fatigue is related to changes in the brain caused by the injury. This student now has to work harder to think and to learn. Work that used to be easy may now be harder and take longer. All this contributes to cognitive and physical fatigue.

The student may look pale and drawn, complain of being tired, frequently yawn, tune out, or even doze off during class. The student may stop to rest in the midst of physical activities or in the middle of an assignment requiring concentration.

Signs to look for...

- ☐ Length of time since injury and return to school
- ☐ Time of day student is most affected by fatigue
- ☐ Cumulative effects of fatigue during school week
- ☐ Length of school day when bus ride is added.
- ☐ Side effects of medications upon attention and energy level
- ☐ Changes in sleep patterns or nightmares
- ☐ Physical limitations which require more effort from student

Changes to consider...

- ☐ Shorten the school day.
- ☐ Provide a break or rest period during school day.
- ☐ Arrange schedule so most difficult work is done when student has most energy.
- ☐ Encourage parents to discuss side effects of medications with physician.

Example

Susan was hospitalized for 17 weeks after being hit by a car while riding her bicycle. When she went home, she still tired easily and napped each afternoon. It was 8 more weeks before she returned to school. During this time a tutor came to her home daily for 2 hours. When she returned to school full time, her teachers noted that she looked tired and pale by mid week. Frequently she chose to remain in her home room during recess. During study periods, she often laid her head on her desk and napped.

Intervention

Despite the appearance of physical well-being, Susan simply had not regained her physical stamina and endurance. Her school day was shortened for the next 3 months. She returned home for lunch, had a short nap or rest period and then finished her school work with a home tutor for one and a half hours.

Irritability and anger

Changes in the student's ability to control emotions may result in sudden temper flare-ups, yelling or swearing outbursts, even hitting or punching others. These changes can frighten teachers and peers, alienate friends and lead to social rejection and isolation. These behaviors may be more frequent when noise and activity levels increase or during stressful situations. Often, the outburst will be brief but intense.

Agitation and irritability are usually the result of fatigue and frustration along with altered ability to control emotions. This behavior can be directly related to damage to the frontal lobes of the brain, but the student's frustration over altered abilities may also cause an emotional reaction. It may be a combination of neurological changes and emotional reactions. It can also be caused by overstimulation in the student's environment.

Signs to look for...

- ☐ Activities that precede irritability or outbursts (called antecedents)
- ☐ Effects of noise and activity on behavior
- ☐ Places where irritability and angry outbursts typically occur
- ☐ Greater frequency of outbursts during certain activities or with particular teachers or classmates
- ☐ Emotional reaction to changes since the injury
- ☐ Degree to which the student is aware of effects of this behavior on others

Changes to consider

- ☐ Track irritability and anger over several weeks to identify causes, frequency and consequences of behaviors.

- ☐ Avoid focusing on the consequences of the behavior and pay more attention to the antecedents. Once the antecedents are identified, modify the environment to avoid triggers.

- ☐ Consult with a neuropsychologist about how to manage and respond to the student's emotional outbursts.

- ☐ Avoid arguing with the student; redirect the student by refocusing the student's attention on something positive.

- ☐ Give feedback on the behavior, but try to avoid punishing the student for behavior that may have been caused by changes in the emotional control centers of the brain.

Example

Tom's quick temper was a constant source of irritation to his teacher. She never knew when he was going to explode when she corrected him for errors in class. He frequently threw his papers on the floor or accused her of picking on him unfairly.

Intervention

The teacher kept a record of Tom's temper outbursts for 2 weeks and noted that they happened most often during math class. Although he received passing grades on his written homework, he had trouble completing math problems on the blackboard during class exercises. With the added pressure of his classmates observing, Tom couldn't concentrate to follow verbal instructions. He became frustrated and embarrassed when he made mistakes and thought other students made fun of him.

The teacher figured out that Tom's trouble following verbal instructions increased under the pressure of classmates watching. When given written instructions to bring to the blackboard, his errors decreased and so did his irritability.

Aggressive acting out or misbehaving

The student hits others, swears, is rude, gets into arguments and disobeys rules. Aggression usually follows a period of agitation. This behavior needs immediate attention because it quickly can result in punishment by teachers and loss of friends. It is especially important that both the family and school staff discuss the relationship of the brain injury and the behavior with a neuropsychologist. Too often, a student is mistakenly labeled as a troublemaker at school and punished when the underlying problem is difficulty controlling feelings and frustrations due to the brain injury. This can compound a student's lowered self-esteem and the belief that, "I can't do anything right" when punished by detention or suspension. Once the downward spiral of lowered self-esteem begins, it can lead to serious depression and/or aggressive outbursts.

Signs to look for

- ☐ History of these behaviors before the injury
- ☐ Activities or environmental changes that are antecedents to behaviors
- ☐ Response of teachers when the student disrupts the class and disturbs others
- ☐ Behaviors in response to the student's frustration with changed cognitive abilities
- ☐ More frequent occurrence with certain teachers or peers
- ☐ Places where outbursts often occur
- ☐ Effects of transitions or changes in routine

Changes to consider

- ☐ Provide more individual attention to reduce frustration that leads to agitation and aggression.
- ☐ Use smaller, more structured setting to reduce triggers or antecedents.
- ☐ Offer an alternative action, for example, take the student for a walk, go to another area, or have the student do something physical to work off frustration.
- ☐ Stay calm; avoid arguing and be a role model for students as you respond.
- ☐ In a confrontation, don't say no; offer a choice or alternative option.
- ☐ Follow emergency procedures if the student's aggressive behavior can not be controlled or threatens the safety of staff or students.

Example

Peter was being sent to the middle school principal's office constantly for punching or hitting classmates. While he had never been the perfect student before his injury, now he was quickly gaining the reputation of troublemaker. Detention was having no effect. Peter was unable to give any reasons for his increasingly frequent fights. A guidance counselor noted that episodes happened most often in the hallways, during gym classes and on the school bus. Unsupervised or unstructured settings with large amounts of noise and activity seemed to overwhelm him and trigger his frustration.

Intervention

Consultation with the neuropsychologist revealed that since his brain injury, Peter quickly became anxious and overstimulated in group situations when noise and activity levels were high. When pushed or shoved in the crowded hallway or school bus, he responded by kicking or punching. Arrangements were made for Peter to change classes five minutes early to minimize time in crowded hallways. The school bus driver reserved a front seat for him. Setting up this structure helped decrease the noise, crowds and confusion that Peter had trouble handling. This helped him feel more in control and fights became less frequent.

Passive behavior

The student "doesn't start anything on his own," or just sits there, "staring off into space." Unmotivated and lazy are words that are often used to describe this student. Unlike the student who constantly gets into trouble, the difficulties of the quiet student may not be noticed as readily. This student easily "slips through the cracks". Passive behavior can be interpreted as not caring when it is actually caused by damage to areas of the brain that control initiating and planning behavior. Once this student gets started, productivity is possible but a structured pathway is needed.

Signs to look for

- ☐ Slow starting an activity
- ☐ Difficulty completing a task
- ☐ Things that help the student get started in an activity

Changes to consider

- ☐ Determine effectiveness of written vs verbal prompts or cues.
- ☐ Use prompts or cues that help this student when stuck.
- ☐ Have a backup system for cuing when the teacher is unavailable.
- ☐ Use a notebook with instructions in words or pictures as cues or reminders
- ☐ Tape cues or reminders on the student's desk for self-prompting
- ☐ Identify and use reinforcers to encourage the student to get through the task.
- ☐ Routinely use a buddy system for cuing

Example

Amy seemed to day dream constantly in class. She listened well and was polite, but she just couldn't seem to keep herself organized. Her teacher and parents were becoming frustrated because she had to be reminded of "every little thing" or else her homework never got done or returned to class. The medical reports noted that due to her brain injury, Amy's ability to initiate or self-prompt was severely limited. She needed cues to help her start activities, but the teacher simply didn't have the time to lead her every step of the way in a class with 23 other students.

Intervention

Amy was given a notebook with critical checkpoints. This was organized by activities where she most frequently got stuck. For example, under the heading End of Homework, there was a checklist for each subject; a place to write assigned pages, chapters, or problems; a section for the day and time the assignment was due; a place to check when the work was done, and a place to check that the completed work was placed in the section marked Completed Work to Bring Back to School.

Depression

Feelings of sadness and loss are normal reactions to a brain injury. They may even be positive signs that the student is aware of changes caused by the injury and is trying to adjust. However, if a student shows or expresses a deep sense of sadness for a long time and makes statements that reflect a loss of self-worth or interest in life, then this is cause for serious concern. Any statements about death or suicide must be taken seriously regardless of the student's age.

It is important to determine the reasons for depression, particularly to sort out the emotional and physical causes. Depression can be caused by direct injury to the brain resulting in altered emotional functioning. Some medications can contribute to depression as well. Many times depression comes from the student feeling or being changed, not being the same person anymore. It can also come from the student's recognition that former goals, hopes and dreams are no longer achievable. A neuropsychologist, psychiatrist or physician experienced in children with brain injuries can evaluate this and design a treatment plan. Social workers and counselors can provide valuable support and counseling. Depression can become a serious and even life threatening condition if ignored.

Sometimes depression is directly related to how the student was injured. For example, motor vehicle crashes often involve others either as passengers or pedestrians. So it is important to know if others were injured or killed and whether friends or relatives were involved. Guilt over the accident and injury is a powerful force that can lead to depression. If the student was hospitalized or unable to attend the funeral of a friend or relative, the mourning process may be delayed and emerge via depression later.

Signs to looks for

- ☐ Changes in sleeping patterns
- ☐ Changes in eating habits
- ☐ Weight gain or loss
- ☐ Loss of interest in usual activities
- ☐ Withdrawal from friends and activities
- ☐ Feelings of hopelessness and that life is not worth living
- ☐ Statements or references about suicide

Changes to consider

- ☐ Meet with parents to learn more about the injury and the student's progress and adjustment.

- ☐ Talk with parents about a referral for a mental health evaluation with a psychiatrist, psychologist or social worker experienced in brain injury.
- ☐ Provide counseling and support. Find opportunities to promote the student's strengths and preferences.
- ☐ Look for a support group for parents and youths via your Brain Injury Association chapter/organization.
- ☐ Develop a peer support network at school.
- ☐ Provide outlets for the student to express feelings via music, writing, or art.
- ☐ Never underestimate the importance of references to suicide or self-destruction.

Example

Susan expressed little interest in her school work and was receiving lower grades in almost every subject. This was in marked contrast to her achievements prior to her injury. She avoided involvement in after school programs and spent little time with her friends at school. Not knowing what to make of her behavior, her friends were at first puzzled, then felt rejected and finally began avoiding her. A referral was made to the school social worker.

Intervention

The social worker called her parents and set up an appointment to meet. Her parents admitted that they also were very worried since she kept to herself at home, shut herself in her room for hours, was eating poorly and having frequent nightmares. They said her older sister had been killed in the same accident just after picking her up from basketball practice. The car was hit by a drunk driver just two blocks from home.

Counseling with Susan revealed that she felt responsible for her sister's death. This was reinforced by her parents' devastating grief and isolation which Susan misinterpreted as anger and rejection. This family needed months of counseling to be able to talk about their losses without feeling overwhelmed. Susan felt guilty because she had survived and needed professional help to overcome these feelings.

With permission, the school social worker shared the cause of Susan's depression with her teachers who gave her extra attention and support during this difficult period.

Teachers effectively used art and poetry to help Susan express her feelings of loss and confusion. They were especially sensitive to her desires about whether she wished to have these shared with her class and family. As she used this method to release some of the emotional tension pent up inside, teachers noted that she gradually emerged from her protective shell and self-imposed seclusion.

Social immaturity

The student's skills for getting along with peers and classmates, acting like others of similar age, making comments that fit the situation and interpreting the reactions and body language of others are generally described as social skills. Sometimes a brain injury affects these skills and the student has less mature behaviors than prior to the injury. Classmates may mimic or make fun of this student because these behaviors seem "babyish." Adolescent peers may find these social breaches embarrassing and reject or avoid the student. This student may need helping relearning social skills just as physical skills like walking or dressing had to be relearned.

Signs to look for

- ☐ Seems stuck at an earlier developmental stage
- ☐ Constant interruptions while others are talking
- ☐ Inability to wait for attention or need to do it RIGHT NOW

- ☐ Frequent tactless remarks
- ☐ Repetition of words or actions like a stuck record
- ☐ Childlike or messy eating habits
- ☐ Difficulty with appropriate dressing or appearance
- ☐ Missed cues during conversations or difficulty interpreting body language
- ☐ Increase in immature behaviors when nervous, anxious or tired

Changes to consider

- ☐ Give direct feedback on social skills to the student and model age appropriate social behavior in real life situations.
- ☐ Talk with peers about cause of altered social skills.
- ☐ Design activities that will include the student with peers to reduce isolation.

Example

Tom's behaviors when he returned to school seemed more typical of a 6 year old than a 3rd grader. His habitual jokes, interruptions during class, and drumming on his desk were especially annoying. The teacher's frustration delighted his classmates who further encouraged him.

Intervention

Tom's ability to monitor his behavior and judge its appropriateness to the situation had been damaged. He reveled in the attention when classmates laughed at his jokes and egged him on when he annoyed the teacher. He not only needed the teacher to establish limits for him by telling him firmly when to stop, but he also needed the teacher's help to channel his energy into other activities that were appropriate for the classroom. Distributing and collecting special supplies, such as chalk or crayons, for special projects, was a more productive way of using his energy and interacting with classmates. No jokes were allowed during class time.

Sexually inappropriate behavior

The brain controls hormonal activity as well as the ability to control and filter our sexual thoughts and actions. When the frontal lobe is damaged, the student may not be able to inhibit sexual urges and may make comments or gestures that are embarrassing to others. As the hormones of adolescence kick in, controlling these impulses may be even more difficult. This behavior can be especially upsetting and embarrassing for parents and friends. Teachers and other students may be insulted, puzzled, or shocked by these sexual comments, or actions. Parents and school staff often worry that such behaviors could lead to sexual intercourse or abuse by peers or strangers.

Signs to look for

- ☐ Verbal comments that are overtly sexual and not appropriate for the situation
- ☐ Physical gestures such as excessive touching or hugging
- ☐ Self stimulation in public
- ☐ Suggestive dressing and appearance
- ☐ Personal or sexual comments or questions to strangers or acquaintances
- ☐ Reactions of peers via encouragement or avoidance

Changes to consider

- ☐ Give direct feedback about what is acceptable and not acceptable in the school setting when inappropriate sexual gestures or comments occur.

- ☐ Help the student learn to self-monitor sexual comments and gestures and track progress daily and/or weekly.

- ☐ Counsel student on possible consequences of sexual behaviors.

- ☐ Consult with a professional to design a behavior management program on sexual behaviors.

- ☐ Work with close peers to develop a buddy system for ongoing feedback outside the classroom to reduce dating and social risks.

- ☐ Coordinate any efforts with parents for reinforcement at home.

Example

When Alison returned to high school after her injury, she approached male classmates for rides , asked them for dates, and made suggestive remarks. Prior to her injury she had been a shy person with limited dating experience. Her friends were embarrassed for her. Those who knew her prior to the accident were cautious and puzzled, and feared that she could "really get into trouble." Others thought she was really "hot" and encouraged her.

Intervention

The guidance counselor met with Alison's closest friends to explain that these changed behaviors were related to her brain injury. Her closest friends became her allies and formed a buddy system while she was at school. They quietly spread the word among her peers that she was still recovering from her injury, that her suggestive remarks and behaviors were not to be treated as jokes or encouraged. The counselor also met with Alison to explain and reinforce the possible consequences of her sexual behaviors.

Forgetfulness

Difficulty with memory and forgetfulness are common and may be temporary or continue over time. Problems with short-term memory are most common. By comparison, long-term memory is often intact after a brain injury. There are numerous aids and techniques to assist individuals with memory problems.

Signs to look for

- ☐ Specific information the student tends to forget
- ☐ Difficulty with subjects, such as history, that require memorization of dates, places and events.
- ☐ Difficulty retrieving recently learned information
- ☐ Confusion over factual information such as places, names, activities, events or dates
- ☐ Repeatedly asking the same questions
- ☐ More difficulty with memory under pressure, when excited or tired
- ☐ Constantly late or mixing up the schedule or classroom locations

Changes to consider

- ☐ Ask parents to identify reminders or prompts that are effective at home and integrate them into the system at school.
- ☐ Develop a written cueing system for use in the classroom and for homework
- ☐ Coordinate cueing system with all teachers and staff
- ☐ Design verbal prompts to help the student remember tasks and assignments
- ☐ Develop a personal notebook or day planner with checklists to help student learn how to self-cue

Example

Bruce's forgetfulness at school constantly resulted in mix-ups and tardiness. Some days were worse than others.

Intervention

Bruce was given a loose leaf notebook to record info and remind him of important activities. There were sections set up for each day, week and month. At the beginning of each day, he reviewed his daily schedule with his home room teacher. It identified any special activities, assignments or events for that day, including the time, place and person in charge. Whenever he became mixed up or confused he referred to his notebook. The teacher made sure that he wrote down all homework assignments or special requests. Changes in schedule, messages for his parents, and special requests were recorded. Due dates for items such as lunch money, recreational school trips, or special events were all listed. A checklist was included for the end of each day to insure that all materials were gathered for the evening's homework assignments before leaving school. An extra set of textbooks were provided for home so that he did not have to remember to carry his books back and forth to school.

Distractibility

Typical consequences of distractibility and difficulty sustaining attention are incomplete assignments and unfinished tasks. The student's concentration is easily interrupted by noise or activity.

Signs to look for

- ☐ Easily distracted by activity in hall, outside windows or other classmates
- ☐ Can't keep up in group activities

- ☐ Improved performance with individual assistance or in small groups
- ☐ Jumps from one topic or activity to another, rarely finishing a task or thought

Changes to consider

- ☐ Provide individual assistance with an aide or tutor to reinforce attention
- ☐ Use small rather than large group activities
- ☐ Break assignments into shorter tasks
- ☐ Move seat to front center row to reduce distractions
- ☐ Clear desktop except for materials needed
- ☐ Modify length of assignments or exercises.
- ☐ Use study corrals in home room, library or at home.

Example

Mary simply couldn't seem to concentrate long enough to finish anything in class. She understood the instructions and was capable of doing the work, but it just didn't get done most of the time.

Intervention

By moving her seat from the outside row near the window to the front of the room by the teacher, Mary was less distracted by noise and activity and better able to concentrate.

Poor organizational skills

This student finds it hard to organize information in terms of priority or will have difficulty completing multistep tasks, such as, "Take out your math book, open to page 83, and do problems 1-20." The student may get the math book out, but not know what to do next. Problems with executive skills like these often result in late or incomplete school assignments.

Signs to look for

- ☐ More trouble with multistep task than one step activities
- ☐ Things are done out of order
- ☐ Student needs more time to get work done
- ☐ Student is regularly behind in class assignments and homework

Changes to consider

- ☐ Give the student a written plan for each school day or have the student write the plan before the day begins
- ☐ Break down instructions into smaller steps
- ☐ Have student review or repeat directions before starting each new step
- ☐ Use verbal or written prompts to help student stay on task
- ☐ Encourage the student to use a signal to alert the teacher when confused about what to do next
- ☐ Design a backup system to use when a teacher is not available
- ☐ Explain the organizational methods used with the student in the classroom to parents so they can use the same methods at home when helping with assignments
- ☐ Develop a buddy system as the student is able to receive assistance from peers when needed

Example

No matter how hard he tried, Kevin got mixed up when the teacher gave instructions unless they were written down. As a result, his work was often incomplete or filled with errors. While others were busy working, Kevin was still trying to sort out the instructions and usually ran out of time. As a result, he was close to failing many subjects.

Intervention

The teacher set up a signal with Kevin that meant he was to wait before starting the exercise. The teacher then broke down the instructions into several mini steps and wrote them down for him to follow. He was given extra time to finish since others started ahead of him.

A final note

This section has described typical changes among students with brain injuries. They are not mutually exclusive; many changes interact with or compound others. The combination of physical, cognitive, emotional, social and behavioral changes are unique for each student. Below is a checklist of possible changes a student might experience following a brain injury.

Physical changes

- ☐ fatigue
- ☐ decreased motor speed and coordination
- ☐ hearing and vision changes
- ☐ headaches

Cognitive changes

- ☐ receptive and expressive language impairments
- ☐ shortened attention and concentration
- ☐ poor memory
- ☐ organizational difficulties

- ☐ difficulty with problem-solving
- ☐ passiveness or slow initiation
- ☐ difficulty sequencing
- ☐ poor self-monitoring
- ☐ impulsiveness

Emotional changes

- ☐ loss of self
- ☐ depression
- ☐ mood swings
- ☐ anxiety

Social and Behavioral changes

- ☐ decreased inhibition
- ☐ decreased judgment
- ☐ aggressiveness
- ☐ difficulty reading social cues
- ☐ self-centeredness
- ☐ lack of confidence
- ☐ withdrawal
- ☐ loss of friends

Assessment and evaluation methods are not exact. Trial and error and common sense approaches by teachers and families often provide the key to effective methods for learning. The next chapter provides more detail on teaching strategies.

Chapter 4
Classroom Strategies
Responding to Student Changes

Parents describe a variety of changes and adjustments after their child has sustained a brain injury. But when asked about the long term challenges they face as a family, school reentry is frequently at the top of the list. Although some children can recover from brain injuries with little or no apparent problems, others return to school and present an entirely different personality, as well as learning style and abilities. This can be puzzling and sometimes frustrating to students in the classroom and to the teacher if careful preparation and planning are not done prior to the student's return. This preparation should include educating the students and the teacher about brain injury.

Many teachers have received little, if any, instruction about brain injury in their course work and feel overwhelmed and unsure of what to expect. Inappropriate expectations for these students can lead to behavior problems and disruption for the entire classroom. After a difficult day at school, the student may have less tolerance for everyday activities at home and may unleash pent up frustrations on family members. Many parents report that their children seem overly fatigued and frustrated when they arrive home from school and are less able to cope with family life. This can result in family life being disrupted even more.

The cerebral cortex is the "thinking" part of the brain that is responsible for communication, memory, planning, organization and new learning. There are two halves or hemispheres that contain four lobes. These are the frontal, parietal, temporal and occipatal lobes. Each lobe is located on the left and right side of the brain.

This chapter helps teachers and other school staff identify the common changes and difficulties that students experience after brain injury and provides suggestions for dealing with them.

Frontal lobes

When a child sustains a brain injury due to a trauma or blow to the head, there is usually damage to the frontal and temporal lobes of the brain - simply because of their location and the way the skull is constructed in these regions.

The frontal lobes are responsible for "executive functions," which include inhibiting responses or reactions, initiating responses/reactions and using good judgment and reasoning. They are responsible for organizing and focusing attention. The frontal lobes govern much of what we do and help us make decisions about our actions.

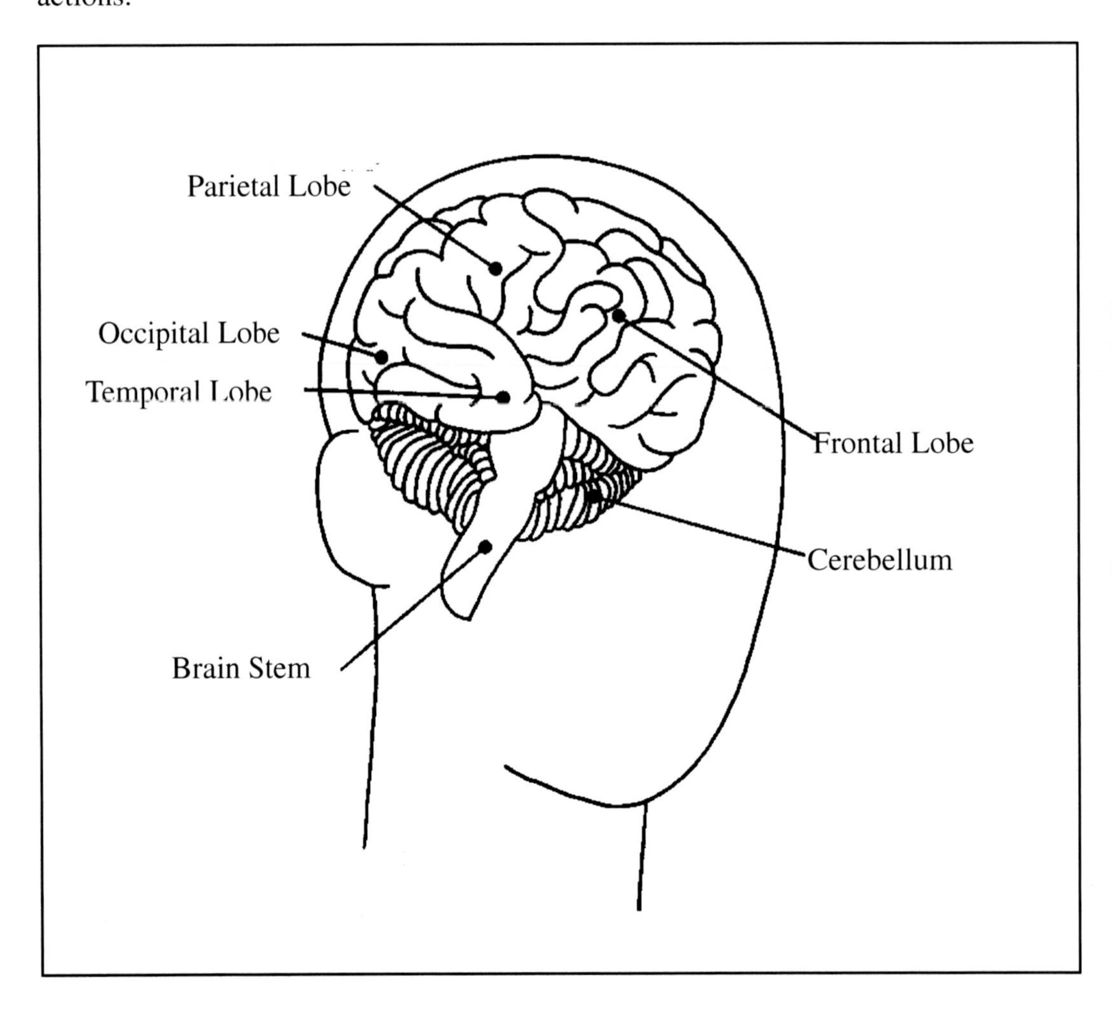

Temporal lobes

The temporal lobes affect emotion, memory and hearing. When the frontal and temporal lobe areas of the brain are injured, it is not surprising to see students having difficulty in the classroom with:

- ☐ attention
- ☐ organization and memory
- ☐ hearing
- ☐ initiating conversation, activities or assignments
- ☐ controlling moods

Occipital lobes

The occipital lobes, located in the back of the head, are responsible primarily for vision. When a person receives a blow to the front of the head (frontal lobes) there can be an opposing force to the back of the head (contra coup) or the occipital lobes, even though the person did not sustain an "outside" injury to that area. An injury to the occipital area may result in damage to the optic nerve and/or limits to the field of vision.

Parietal lobes

The parietal lobes of the brain are involved with touch perception and sensation. Students with damage to this area of the brain may not be able to perceive when they are being touched or when they are touching something or someone. It would, for example, be difficult for students to play an instrument like the violin or piano if they could not watch their fingers. Similarly, these students might have difficulty keyboarding or typing.

Parietal lobe function allows us to reach into a bag or purse and identify a set of keys, a comb or a tube of lipstick by touch alone.

Left and right hemispheres

Students with damage to the left hemisphere of the brain may have more difficulty with language related activities, such as reading and writing, whereas a student with right hemisphere damage may have more difficulty with spatial skills and social perceptions (i.e., reading body language, facial expressions). And yet, one area of the brain never works in isolation from the others; they are connected in countless ways, many of which are yet unknown.

Effects upon students and importance of teachers

Students with brain injuries may have difficulty expressing what they know because of language and/or organizational problems. These students fatigue more easily, and may not have the stamina for a full school day. They may need to work and concentrate much harder to do things they used to do quite easily which can also increase fatigue.

Transitions from one activity to another require more preparation for this student. Many individuals have difficulty dealing with abrupt changes in a routine or schedule - this is a common difficulty for a person with a brain injury. Persons who have survived a brain injury say that the key to their survival and ability to be independent lies in the structure and organization of their day. When this is removed or changed, they become confused and less able to cope and function.

When a person has a traumatic brain injury, it is unlikely that just one area of the brain will be damaged. Teachers must be aware of the many possible effects on a student's learning, social interactions and overall behavior in the classroom. Teachers must also be able to generate ways to assist the student or make adaptations.

Following are some ideas to get started. As you read over the list, you will probably see ideas/techniques that you have used with other students in your classroom over the years; students who need modifications to assist them with their attention, learning, and behavior. It is not necessarily a list of adaptations for students with brain injury - it is a list of ideas that will work with any student who may be experiencing trouble of one kind or another in your classroom. There is nothing magic about the list; the "magic" occurs when you find the idea or strategy that will help put the student's world back into perspective, which will make the days (and nights) easier for everyone to manage.

Fatigue

Some students do not return to school for a full day. If they start by going half days, make sure that it is their best half of the day. If they are slow to get going in the morning, consider afternoon classes. If they opt to take only 1-2 classes, try to ensure that the classes are at a good time of the day and that they are classes that the student was doing well in previously. This can help school reentry get off to a positive start. Whether the student attends for half or full days, make sure that short rest breaks are available throughout the day and provide a place, such as the nurses station, for the student to lie down to rest as needed.

Memory/Organization

Everyone develops methods of organization to get through the day to avoid forgetting or neglecting important things. Assisting a student with organizational strategies may be one of the most helpful things done for the student and family. Many adults use notebooks or calendars to jot down appointments and reminders; this is a good idea for students with memory and organizational difficulties. It is important that the student not be solely responsible for this. Family members and school personnel need to assist the student at the key points listed below.

When	What needs to be done	Who checks
before leaving for school	Is there a list of all the things to be returned to school?	parent
arrival at school	Does the student have everything needed to get started in the morning?	teacher/case manager/aide
end of each class	Are assignments written down in the notebook?	teacher/aide
end of school day	What needs to go home?	teacher/case manager/aide
arrival home	What homework or paperwork needs to be done and returned to school the next day?	parent

- **Extra set of books**

Since it takes extra energy to take books home and bring them back to school, and extra effort to remember them, purchasing an extra set of textbooks for home can be helpful. Important information in the texts can also be highlighted if they are purchased specifically for the student.

- **Backpack**

A backpack is useful for carrying things to and from school, particularly for a student with motor problems. The backpack should be with the student at all times.

- **Written schedule**

A schedule of the day's activities can be taped to the student's desk and inside the organization notebook to help remember the routine and any special activities.

- **Buddy system**

A buddy system can be invaluable to a student with a brain injury. The "buddy" can be one or more students or peers with whom the teacher, the family and the student all feel comfortable. Use of a peer to prompt or remind is less obtrusive than an adult. Continuous intervention by adults usually means that less interaction with peers will occur, which can be detrimental to social skill development. Use of a buddy might also provide needed structure and assistance for the unexpected such as fire drills, weather alerts and other emergency situations.

- **Reduce changes**

Reducing the number of changes in the student's routine will also help a student with organization. As previously mentioned, the "routine" is essential for a student with memory difficulties. Changes in routine may leave the student not knowing what to do or where to go.

Motor difficulties

Students who have residual problems with motor skills may find it difficult to complete written work in the classroom. Motor problems may not allow them to work quickly or efficiently and the finished project may not be legible or accurately reflect their effort.

➢ Help with written tasks

Some students need writing paper stabilized with some masking tape or a piece of dycem (nonskid material used by many occupational therapists). Students whose motor difficulties are more severe can benefit from using a computer for writing and a calculator for math (see math section for more detailed information about the calculator).

➢ Reduce written work

Even these assists may not be sufficient to help a student keep pace with the rest of the class. If this is the case, then other alternatives need to be explored. Consider reducing the written work that is required. For example, writing spelling words in sentences is a frequent assignment. If the goal is for the student to learn how to spell 25 words for the week, then the focus should be on spelling, not sentence construction. If a secondary goal is to improve sentence construction, then perhaps the student could practice writing/typing the words and use 5-10 of them in a sentence, rather than all 25. The end result is that the student: a) learns to spell the words; b) gets some practice with sentence construction, and c) keeps up with the rest of the class.

The same idea can be used in math; rather than having a student copy and complete 30-50 math problems, problems that reflect new math skills could be written out and the teacher could pick 10-20 problems that represent new skills being learned. If the student can demonstrate mastery with those 10-20 problems, it is probably not necessary to complete 50. Class time and effort could be spent learning additional skills; evening time could be spent with the family, rather than on homework assignments.

➢ Use dictation

The buddy system also works well when adapting for motor difficulties, as the "buddy" can become a peer secretary, who writes down dictated responses. This works extremely well for the student who would otherwise take enormous amounts of time to complete written work, even when using a computer or calculator.

Student helpers who volunteer to be a peer secretary must be instructed to write down exactly what the student dictates, regardless of whether it is correct. In this way, the teacher has an accurate picture of the student's abilities and identifies which areas continue to need work. If there is a teacher assistant or volunteer working in the classroom, these individuals can take dictation from the student, who otherwise, might fall behind in written work because of motor problems. The student's knowledge can be checked quickly by asking the student to complete the assignment orally and recording the child's oral performance, just as would be done with written work.

- **Give extra time**

Sometimes a student's motor problems are mild and do not require any specific adaptations, but do require that extra time be given to complete assignments. Arrange study halls after classes that consistently require written work (Literature, English, Math); or provide assistance from a teacher aide, peer or resource teacher near the end of the school day. But bear in mind that providing assistance at the end of the school day may not be effective for students who are fatigued by that time. They need assistance earlier in the day.

Last of all, if you know that a student works more slowly than the average student, try to avoid timed tests and other activities. They will not provide an accurate picture of this child's abilities and knowledge. (See note taking in next section)

Reading

If a student had learning problems prior to the injury, it is possible that the problems will be more pronounced afterward. In reading, inefficient word decoding skills and/or a slower reading rate contribute to a student's inability to comprehend material and keep pace with the rest of the class.

- **Use audio books**

Audio books are readily available for text books and leisure reading materials through many state associations for persons with visual impairments. In addition, many of these organizations can provide recorded materials for persons with physical impairments and reading disabilities. The student with reading problems can follow along in the text while listening to the recording on a set of headphones, while other students in the class are reading the material. Leisure reading material (audio version) encourages the student to listen to the same books that peers are reading, which contributes to an increase in general knowledge and age appropriate information. Discussion of the book with peers may also assist the student in social interactions.

- **Adapt tests**

Students with reading difficulties need to have adaptations made when they are required to take (read) tests. Test can be administered orally by a teacher aide or adult volunteer and the student can provide oral answers since writing skills are usually weaker than reading skills.

- **Help with note taking**

A student with weak reading/writing skills will also need assistance in classes which require note taking. Important text information can be highlighted in the student's personal text books; probably the most helpful assist, however, is a carbon or xerox copy of another student's notes. The process should be discussed ahead of time with both students, so that they are willing participants. Documentation of this and other adaptations in the student's educational program (IEP) is a good idea for future teachers. Discussing it with the parents of both students is also suggested. Although the student may need help reading notes, they will serve as a study guide and a summary for the student and others working with him prior to taking a test.

- **Give extra instruction**

A student with a reading disability can often benefit from remedial reading instruction. Memory problems can interfere, however, with the ability to utilize typical approaches to reading that incorporate the use of phonics, blending sounds and the memorization of sight words. If this is the case, the instructor might try to teach reading by "chunking information" or using word families such as fight, right, sight, light, etc.

Math

Students with reading disabilities or memory problems will often have difficulty with the memorization of basic math facts. Certainly, a teacher will want to continue working on these with the student, but not to the point where the student falls hopelessly behind the rest of the class. Whether a student counts on fingers, uses a math fact sheet, practices with flashcards or uses a calculator, the end result is the same; the student sees the correct answer and tries to commit it to memory. Once a student is sure of the answer, time will not be wasted using the calculator or counting fingers; the student will simply write it down. On the other hand, if the student is unable to commit these facts to memory, you have provided an appropriate alternative to use when there is no one around to help.

- **Use a calculator**

This becomes especially important as students reach adolescence and need a reliable alternative for dealing with math in activities of daily living (going to the movie, the store, or out for pizza with friends). In this day and age, it is not unusual to see someone using a calculator - at any age. If, after several years of instruction, a student is still experiencing problems with math facts, it would be a wiser use of teacher and student time to place more emphasis on teaching functional calculator skills. Primarily, this involves the use of story problems (written or oral) so that the student learns how and when to use certain operations, particularly for math in activities of daily living.

One final word about math and calculators - the calculator is also useful and sometimes necessary for a student with a physical impairment. Even though a student may show good potential for memorizing math facts, if the physical impairment is severe enough to significantly affect a student's work rate and written work is difficult to read, then use of a calculator may be more appropriate. Ask yourself, "How will this student function most appropriately, efficiently and accurately when dealing with math as an adult?" If motor skills will interfere with math performance, shouldn't we provide instruction that will allow the student to function in "the least restrictive" but most productive and satisfying way as an adult?

Social Skills

Use of a buddy system for redeveloping social skills can be helpful, particularly in unstructured situations (playground, hallway, lunchroom) where the student may be prone to having difficulty. Again, continual intervention by an adult may draw unwanted attention to the student and can discourage peers from interacting.

➢ Organize a buddy system

A "buddy" can redirect, prompt and cue less obtrusively than an adult. When using the buddy system, it may be helpful/necessary to utilize several students so that no one student feels overly responsible. It is also important to choose students who genuinely care about their classmate and are interested in working through the difficulties. As always, it is a good idea to notify the parents of all students involved so that they have knowledge and understanding of these activities. Since unstructured activities tend to create problems for many students with brain injuries, it is wise for school personnel to increase supervision in these areas, at least initially, to ensure the safety of the student and to intervene if necessary.

➢ Use real life situations

When trying to develop or improve social relationships and interactions, try to use real life situations rather than setting up something artificial. This is more meaningful for the student. For example, sitting with a small group of students at lunch (which many students use as a social time) may provide insight as to where problems occur. There are certainly other students within the classroom or school who could also benefit from social skills feedback in a group like this. A "buddy" or case manager may be able to provide helpful suggestions to the student during lunch or immediately following. Special clubs or groups may also provide opportunities to interact; teachers involved need to communicate with each other in order to identify areas which need work and to identify areas that are improving.

➢ Coordinate and communicate

A case manager or social worker for the student can help coordinate efforts and communication between the family, school and medical personnel. The case manager can also serve as a "counselor" for the student when necessary. There may be times when the student feels overwhelmed, frustrated, embarrassed or angry and needs a safe place to go and a trusted person with whom to talk. The case manager can also keep other professionals informed of the student's feelings and specific areas of difficulty.

Attention

A student's ability to pay attention, especially for extended periods of time, may be impaired after a brain injury.

➢ Shorten assignments

Provide shorter assignments, or break them down into smaller tasks to help the student maintain attention. Many adults find that they are able to attend better to material if they take short breaks. Some students find it motivating to work with a timer, i.e., "See how much of this you can finish before the timer rings... you will receive extra points...or I will give you a break...or you will receive a sticker...or you can listen to music on your walkman for five minutes." The ideas can be as varied as your imagination and knowledge of what motivates the student.

➢ Minimize distractions

Most individuals have to cope with distractions as they work; noises, conversations, activity in the room or out the window. The student with attention problems may find that a quiet corner of the room or a study carrel will help reduce these distractions. Some individuals are better able to focus if there is "white noise" or soft music in the background. This can be accomplished easily in the classroom by providing the student with a tape and a set of headphones.

Behavior

Parents and teachers identify behavior problems as a major concern after a brain injury. Some students may not perceive or understand the changes in their performance and other students are painfully aware of the abilities and skills that have been lost. At any rate, there are some things to keep in mind to avoid or minimize the problems that occur.

➢ Avoid changes in routine

Routine and structure are critical to a student with memory problems. Changes in routine may increase the student's confusion and disorganization. On the other hand, we live in a world where change is constant and things are not always predictable, so when a change in routine is necessary, provide as much transition time as possible to help the student get ready mentally. Offer an explanation for the change and enlist the student's help. For example, "We are going next door for a movie instead of going outside because the weather is bad. Will you help me by taking the videotape over to Ms. Smith's room?" Or, whenever possible, remind the student, "In five minutes, we will be leaving for science class."

➢ Give choices

It also helps to give the student choices to provide them with a sense of control over their life and activities. For example, "We won't be able to go outside today because the weather is bad - would you like to watch a video with Ms. Smith's class, listen to your Walkman or use the computer in our classroom?"

Giving choices can also be helpful in terms of completing assignments, i.e., "You need to finish your spelling words and complete the math problems in your workbook. Which would you like to tackle first?" Giving choices and providing transitions may help avoid power struggles with the student.

➢ Be flexible

Don't be afraid to change or reduce expectations if they seem unrealistic or if the student is consistently unsuccessful. It doesn't mean that you've "given in" or lost the battle - only that you've made an attempt to help the student experience success. Most individuals will find ways to avoid work that is too difficult and no one wants to experience failure over and over. Adults want to be successful at work; school *is* the student's work.

➢ Adjust schedule

Behavior problems can become more pronounced when the student is tired and feels ill-equipped to handle an assignment or activity. Try to assign difficult classes earlier in the day or at a time when the student is more alert. Initiating, problem solving and attending will all be easier if the student is rested and alert.

➢ Use a diary

A diary provides the student with an additional outlet. It gives the student a place to record feelings, thoughts and reactions. With the student's permission, it may provide some insight to parents and professionals about the student's world. These thoughts and feelings can be discussed with a specific teacher, case manager, counselor, or parent so that the student receives some feedback and closure.

The diary can also be used to describe incidents that occur during the day (bad ones and good ones) so that these can be used as examples to the student in shaping future behavior, i.e., "What else could you have done or said to avoid this conflict?" or "What do you think it was that you said or did that helped this situation?" Remember, if you decide to use a diary, the student may need help recording and organizing thoughts and ideas.

A final comment

It is important to focus on the concept or skill that you want the student to learn and to find the most efficient, effective (and fun!) route to the mastery of that concept. This saves the student's time and energy and avoids frustration for both student and teacher.

Chapter 5
Working with the Neuropsychologist

Neuropsychologists have special training to evaluate how a brain injury affects learning, communication, planning, organization and interpersonal relationships. Already trained in psychology, the neuropsychologist specializes in the relationships between the brain and behavior. The neuropsychologist can evaluate how the brain injury affects the student's ability to:

- learn
- communicate
- plan and organize
- relate to others

The neuropsychologist uses a variety of tests (games, puzzles, responses to words and images) to understand how the brain injury affects the student's ability to function. To be a neuropsychologist, one must earn a Ph.D. in psychology and complete specialized training and internships in neuropsychology.

The neuropsychologist is different than a *neurologist* who is a physician that focuses on the physical structure of the brain and nervous system. The neuropsychologist is different than a *psychologist* who has the same basic training, but has not specialized in neuropsychology. A psychologist may not be able to do the more detailed evaluations needed for a student with a brain injury.

Intelligence and achievement tests (often given by school psychologists) are not always helpful when evaluating a student with a brain injury because significant parts measure what the child has learned in the past. Often a student with a brain injury does not lose the academic knowledge gained prior to injury. Thus, test scores on sections of I.Q. tests which rely on previously learned material (such as vocabulary, general information, social comprehension) often show little or no loss. This can give a misleading picture of the student's ability to function in the classroom and to learn new information. It can contribute to the perception of the student as "lazy" or "unmotivated".

The neuropsychologist can help parents and teachers...

- ☐ identify how the student learns and uses new information
- ☐ understand changes in behavior
- ☐ design compensatory strategies
- ☐ develop an educational program
- ☐ identify changes to watch for as the child matures and progresses through school
- ☐ obtain baseline information and chart the student's progress over time

When to ask for a neuropsychological evaluation

There is no set timetable for a neuropsychological evaluation. The brain changes rapidly during the first year after the injury. Many students experience new challenges with each developmental milestone as latent effects emerge. Indicators that an evaluation is needed are...

- ☐ When information is needed about a student's present level of performance
- ☐ When a student has acquired a moderate to severe brain injury
- ☐ When a student has sustained a mild traumatic brain injury or concussion and is still having trouble with attention, learning, behavior or emotions after several months
- ☐ Lowered grades and new or additional difficulties with learning
- ☐ Behaviors interfere with learning at school and interpersonal relationships
- ☐ Any time significant problems or changes in functioning arise that educators and parents cannot explain or work with effectively

When you hear comments such as:

PARENT	"He's failing and I don't understand why!"
TEACHER	"I've tried everything in class and nothing seems to work!"
TEAM	"He does well in some situations, but terribly in others!"

These are signs that it is time to involve a neuropsychologist to help define the problem and develop strategies to help the student. If the child is still in a rehabilitation program, ask that a neuropsychological evaluation be done before the child is discharged in order to have a baseline for later comparison. Parents should keep copies of these reports and also provide them to the educational team as part of the eligibility determination process for special education.

Methods of evaluation

A formal evaluation involves hours of testing, observation and interviews that enable the examiner to develop both detailed information and data as well as a general impression of the student's abilities. Evaluations usually involve tests that use games, puzzles, and responses that are designed to give the examiner information about how different parts of the student's brain function when challenged to reason, analyze, store and recall information. The selection of which tests are administered depends on the student's age, reported difficulties and the information that is being requested. Therefore, it's important to carefully prepare the request so that the examiner selects the instruments that will address the areas where the student is having difficulty.

There are also informal methods of assessment that can be used. The neuropsychologist may be asked to...

- ☐ review the student's medical and educational records
- ☐ provide an in-service on brain injury for the educational team and staff
- ☐ observe the student in the classroom
- ☐ meet with the parents and educational team
- ☐ consult and problem solve on an ongoing basis or as needed

How to select a neuropsychologist

The school district may have an ongoing contract with a neuropsychologist. If a neuropsychologist has not been identified or previously used, consider looking for recommendations from the state's professional psychology association or the state chapter of the Brain Injury Association. Other local schools in the region or district may have identified other students with brain injuries and give recommendations on neuropsychologists they have used and found effective. Local rehabilitation providers may also be able to give recommendations.

Ask if the neuropsychologist has experience with...

- ☐ children
- ☐ age of the child or student
- ☐ current stage of student's recovery or length of time post injury
- ☐ schools and special education programs
- ☐ designing and recommending compensatory strategies and instructional strategies for the classroom

What to share with the neuropsychologist

Making the referral is not the responsibility of only one person. It is a three way process between parents, educators and the neuropsychologist. Parents and educators need to be clear about what they are requesting, the difficulties that they are having, what information is needed, and their expectations for follow-up. The neuropsychologist needs to be clear about what information can be provided, how the results will be communicated and interpreted, and the implications of the test results for the student's learning and instruction.

By providing the neuropsychologist with as much information as possible during the referral process, the examiner can determine which tests will provide the information that the school and family needs. Assuming that the neuropsychologist will somehow "know what to do" makes the job much more difficult. Remember, that the parents and educational team have extensive knowledge and observation of the student that is valuable and needs to be shared with the examiner in order for the evaluation to be effective.

Parents can provide information on...

- ☐ date and cause of injury
- ☐ history of medical and rehabilitation care
- ☐ current medications and/or medical treatments
- ☐ summary of student's strengths and weaknesses prior to injury
- ☐ changes in abilities, behaviors and learning after the injury
- ☐ concerns about their child's education
- ☐ questions about their child's future

Educators can provide ...

- ☐ A list of concerns, questions and observations about the student's strengths and needs.
- ☐ Current records of grades and any other information about the student's present and past classroom performance.
- ☐ Any preinjury results from standardized tests or formal assessments.
- ☐ A description of current school programs and activities and a detailed educational history.
- ☐ The student's individualized educational program and quarterly reports if the student is receiving special education services.
- ☐ A completed Worksheet: *Transition Back to School Following Brain Injury.* (See worksheet section of this book)

What to ask the neuropsychologist

There is no preset list of questions to ask; it is different for each student because each brain injury is unique. However, the following list suggests areas to consider.

- ☐ Does this student have a brain injury or does the history indicate that a brain injury occurred although medical documentation is incomplete.

- ☐ How does the brain injury affect the student's
  - work in groups
  - need for individualized instruction
  - ability to learn new materials
  - efforts in timed tests/quizzes
  - control over behavior
  - ability to participate in group social situations
  - social interactions with friends
  - ability to complete assignments on time
  - stamina during school day
  - performance relaated to medications and possible side effects
  - emotional adjustment and sense of well-being

How can teachers work effectively with the student? Ask if the report will...

- ☐ describe the student's current strengths and needs

- ☐ explain the student's most effective learning styles

- ☐ give examples of what teachers can do in the classroom that will emphasize the student's strengths

- ☐ suggest activities where peers can help

- ☐ provide suggestions for parents/family members at home

What will be the most effective way for the neuropsychologist to conduct the evaluation?

☐ visit the school and observe the student in the classroom

☐ watch a video of the student in school or at home in challenging situations

☐ test in office

☐ adjust testing schedule for physical factors such as fatigue and cognitive factors such as shortened attention span or distractibility. Other factors are time of day and distance of travel.

What to get from the neuropsychologist

There are several methods that neuropsychologists use to provide information. Some write lengthy and detailed reports. Some involve colleagues, including therapists and counselors, to supplement reports of test results with detailed narratives of how this data relates to the student's performance and teaching strategies in the classroom. Others provide follow-up consultation to guide educators in the interpretation of the test results and to help them design educational programs. However, it is always preferable to have a written record of findings as well as recommendations for continuity and consistency among the various people working with the student. It is also important to have a means, whether through writing, telephone or consultation, to obtain specific suggestions and techniques for...

☐ classroom strategies to assist student in completing assignments

☐ methods to improve new learning

☐ effective ways to prompt/redirect student

☐ management of inappropriate or difficult behavior

☐ guidelines for learning in various settings
- one-to-one
- small group

☐ use of adaptive devices for memory, communication, organization

- alternative methods of student evaluation
  - open book tests
  - untimed tests
  - oral vs. written
  - pictures vs. words
  - multiple choice vs. essay
  - techniques for reading: silent vs. auditory

Payment for the neuropsychological evaluation

While the cost varies depending on the number of tests administered and the hours required, formal testing, review of records, and report writing can easily be quite expensive. The previous suggestions help insure that the investment is worth it. Two primary methods of payment are through health insurance or under special education. Determining who pays for this often involves discussion over whether it is a medical concern or an educational issue.

A baseline neuropsychological evaluation that is done while the child is still hospitalized or in a rehabilitation program may be covered by the family's health insurance. It is done to help assess the early stages of cognitive recovery from the physical trauma of the injury.

As latent effects of the brain injury emerge in school, the neuropsychological evaluation is both a tool to measure ongoing and long-term brain functioning as well as to assess the effects of the injury upon the student's ability to learn and function in school. Thus, it is based upon the need to gather information about how this student is currently learning, how the injury has affected the student's cognitive abilities, and what educational tools and strategies will help the student learn and function more effectively in school. In this case, payment may be sought through special education funds.

Sometimes, payment is shared by health insurers and special education; thus, reducing the cost to each. This also recognizes that there is a medical and educational component to this testing and evaluation.

A final comment

An initial evaluation prior to or just after the student returns to school creates baseline information which is invaluable in reassessment and educational planning later.

A student will be changing and improving as time goes on, especially in the first year or two after the injury. New difficulties may emerge. Follow-up neuropsychological evaluations may be more effective in assisting with educational planning after the child returns to school.

The information from a neuropsychological evaluation can actually save the school district money by providing critical information for building *effective and efficient* educational plans that directly meet the student's needs.

Example

Tom's grades slipped from a solid B average to C-. The psychologist's report offered no insight as standard testing showed abilities well above average. His grades were particularly puzzling because Tom clearly excelled in some subjects and in others he seemed hopelessly lost. He followed instructions in class, asked good questions, and did his homework. On multiple choice test questions he scored high; however, on essay questions he rambled on with no clear logic or order. He seemed to concentrate on just writing down as much information as he could remember and hoped that some of it answered the question.

Intervention

Any major change or inconsistency in grades following an injury is a sign that difficulties may be related to changes in how the brain functions. Tom's recall and recognition of information was good. This is why he did well on multiple choice tests. It was his ability to conceptualize and draw relationships between cause and effect and to organize information that was damaged, hence, his difficulty with essay tests. By modifying test formats to give him more structured questions, his grades improved.

Worksheet 1
Transition Back to School

Introduction

Because structure and consistency are so important for a student with a brain injury, any change or transition requires special planning. Yet changes constantly occur in school during each day and week as well as over the school year. The student's initial return or entry to school after an injury is just the first of many transitions. This section provides detailed work sheets to help parents and educators prepare the student for the necessary transitions over time.

Lash & Associates Publishing/Training gives permission to copy all of the work sheets in this manual so they can be used by parents and educators.

Initial return to school worksheet

This worksheet is designed to help the educational team plan for the student's return to school. The information needed to complete this worksheet may come from many sources including family members, medical and rehabilitation staff, other educators who have worked with the student in the past, and by direct observation and discussion with the student.

Brain injuries can cause impairments in all areas of the student's cognitive, social/behavioral, and sensorimotor functioning with unique and sometimes unanticipated consequences. Only a holistic look at the student's history, medical/rehabilitative services, and current strengths/needs can reveal the specific pattern of disabilities confronting the student with a brain injury.

Student name ______________________________ **Date** ________________

Age and grade now___________ **Age and grade at time of injury** ___________

1. Description of injury

The events and experiences of a child's injury often have long term emotional consequences that the teacher and guidance counselor should be aware of when working with the student and her/his family.

Date of injury: ____

Describe events leading to student's injury: ___________________________

____

____

____

Describe all physical injuries:___________________________________

____

____

____

In this description, please consider

- ☐ Involvement of family members or close friends?
- ☐ Was someone found to be at fault? Have formal charges been brought?
- ☐ Is there current litigation?
- ☐ Were others injured? Did anyone die?
- ☐ Was alcohol or drug use a factor?

2. Description of family

A brain injury is a traumatic event in the life of a family. The injury, hospitalization/rehabilitation process, and the student's resulting needs and disabilities have a social and emotional impact on each family member. It is an event that often consumes the time, financial, and emotional resources of the entire family.

Family members

Mother ____________________

Father ____________________

Parents are: ☐ married ☐ separated ☐ divorced

Step parent ____________________

Siblings (age, grade in school)

____

____

Others (relationship to student)

____

____

How is the family coping with long term medical or care issues?

____

____

Describe the family's strengths which can be built upon to establish a school-family partnership:

____

____

3. Time frames

Time is an indicator of the length of the student's medical recovery as well as the cumulative stress upon families. Length of coma is an indicator of the severity of the brain injury. More than 24 hours indicates a severe brain injury; more than 1 hour but less than 24 hours indicates a moderate brain injury.

Define time frames

Length of coma # hours_______ # days_______ # weeks_______

Hospital stay admitted_______________ discharged________________

Time in rehabilitation program admitted__________ discharged____________

Outpatient services started_____________ ended_____________

4. Description of medical care & rehabilitation

Define services/contacts/records

Hospital stay	Name	Records rec'd
Physical therapy	________________________________	☐
Speech/Language therapy	________________________________	☐
Occupational therapy	________________________________	☐
Social work	________________________________	☐
Counseling	________________________________	☐
Other	________________________________	☐
Other	________________________________	☐

Rehabilitation program	**Name**	**Records rec'd**
Physical therapy	______________________________	☐
Speech/Language therapy	______________________________	☐
Occupational therapy	______________________________	☐
Neuropsychology/psychology	______________________________	☐
Educational & vocational	______________________________	☐
Social work	______________________________	☐
Other	______________________________	☐

Outpatient services	**Name**	**Records rec'd**
Physical therapy	______________________________	☐
Speech/language therapy	______________________________	☐
Occupational therapy	______________________________	☐
Neuropsychology/psychology	______________________________	☐
Social work	______________________________	☐
Other	______________________________	☐

Describe current medical condition

Medical/nursing care ______________________________

Medications ______________________________

Seizure Activity ______________________________

Assistive Devices ______________________________

Activity restrictions ______________________________

Other ______________________________

5. Description of pre-injury functioning

Developmental history

Delays in early childhood development ____________________________________

Special needs or disabilities prior to injury ________________________________

Prior significant illness/injury ____

Change in right or left handedness ____

School history prior to injury

Achievement Test Scores **Dates Administered**

____

____

____

Reading ___________________________ Grade level performance ____________

Math ______________________________ Grade level performance ____________

Written work _______________________ Grade level performance ____________

Other _____________________________ Grade level performance ____________

History of Spec Ed services ____

____

_________________________________ Date of last plan (IEP) ____________

Name/phone - chair of committee _____________________________________

Name/phone - last teacher(s)____

Name/phone - last teacher(s)____

Involvement in school extra curricular activities

____

____

History of school behavior problems/disciplinary actions (if any)

____

____

Work habits and social interaction

____

____

Social/family functioning

Describe student's pre-injury relationships with family members

____

____

Describe student's pre-injury relationships with classmates and peers

____

____

Activity prior to injury

Employment _______________________________________

Volunteer activities _________________________________

Extra-curricular activities ____________________________

Athletics and sports _________________________________

6. Description of current functioning

Start by checking the student's strengths or difficulties in all categories.

Cognitive-communicative	**✔ Strengths**	**✔ Difficulties**
alertness	☐	☐
response to noise/activity	☐	☐
response to change	☐	☐
attention/concentration	☐	☐
problem solving	☐	☐
speed of thinking/responding	☐	☐
language skills	☐	☐
memory for new information	☐	☐
retrieval of old information	☐	☐
flexibility/adjustment to change	☐	☐
initiating activities	☐	☐
planning ahead	☐	☐
sequencing	☐	☐
completes assignments	☐	☐
follows schedule	☐	☐
functions independently	☐	☐
gets to classes on time	☐	☐
fatigue	☐	☐
impulse control	☐	☐

Academic	✔ **Strengths**	✔ **Difficulties**
grade level performance	☐	☐
reading	☐	☐
math	☐	☐
written work	☐	☐
other ______________________________	☐	☐

Modifications needed	✔ Yes	✔ No	✔ Maybe
altered schedule	☐	☐	☐
length of school day	☐	☐	☐
structured work/activities	☐	☐	☐
frequent breaks	☐	☐	☐
rest period	☐	☐	☐
relocation of instruction/classes	☐	☐	☐
length of assignments	☐	☐	☐
work expectations/speed	☐	☐	☐
alternative testing formats	☐	☐	☐
instructional methods/materials/aids	☐	☐	☐
compensatory strategies	☐	☐	☐
adaptive equipment/technology	☐	☐	☐
organizational systems	☐	☐	☐
communication systems	☐	☐	☐

	✔ Yes	✔ No	✔ Maybe
behavior plans or supports	☐	☐	☐
reinforcers	☐	☐	☐

Social/behavioral	**✔ Strengths**	**✔ Difficulties**
awareness of needs	☐	☐
peer support	☐	☐
interpersonal relationships	☐	☐
awareness of social rules/roles	☐	☐
self care/appearance/grooming	☐	☐
age-appropriate behavior	☐	☐
impulse control	☐	☐
sexuality	☐	☐
mood swings	☐	☐
depression	☐	☐
use of alcohol/drugs	☐	☐
other ____________________________	☐	☐

Sensorimotor	**✔ Strengths**	**✔ Difficulties**
coordination and balance	☐	☐
strength and endurance	☐	☐
mobility	☐	☐
right/left handedness	☐	☐

vision	☐	☐
hearing	☐	☐
spatial orientation	☐	☐
loss of smell	☐	☐
spasticity	☐	☐
numbness or pain	☐	☐
other ___________________________	☐	☐
other ___________________________	☐	☐

7. Description of the student's goals

The personal goals of the student (no matter what age) can be a powerful force leading to change and adaptation. Many times the goals appear to be completely unrealistic and unattainable. Sometimes the injury to the student's brain affects judgment to the degree that the student is unable to understand that a goal is not realistic. However, the goals can offer a clue to the student's interests and can be broken down into achievable steps.

Example

Tom is a high school student with a severe disability from a brain injury. In his junior year in high school, Tom was the star quarterback and planned to play football in college after graduation. Following his injury, he told the guidance counselor that he didn't need vocational counseling because he already knew what he was going to do. He would be the quarterback for the Detroit Lions professional football team. Clearly, this was not possible due to his cognitive and physical injuries.

Tom's parents found his inability to recognize his limitations very distressing. However, school staff focused on Tom's interest and worked with him to define the steps leading to his goal. Building his physical endurance through an exercise program, catching and throwing a ball, writing out and graphing football plays helped to build important skills for Tom. As Tom made progress on his short term objectives, he began to become aware of how difficult it would be to attain his ultimate goal. Over time, he refocused his vocational goal to be a trainer in a health/fitness club.

Identify the student's short term goals

short term - the next 3 to 6 months

over the student's school career

long term as an adult - vocational , residential and community

8. Description of parental/family support

family strengths/resources to cope

insight into child's disability

parental/family goals for student - short term and long term

parental concerns about return to school

family support services/information

9. Summary of initial program

	✔ Yes	✔ No	✔ Maybe
home tutoring	☐	☐	☐
special placement	☐	☐	☐
partial school day	☐	☐	☐
full school day	☐	☐	☐
rest periods	☐	☐	☐
special transportation	☐	☐	☐
general education	☐	☐	☐
other ______________________	☐	☐	☐

Special services

What	When	Who

10. Schedule and planning issues

How will ongoing medical and rehabilitation care be coordinated with the school schedule?

Medication administration (who, when, how?)

Outside medical appointments

Special transportation arrangements

Worksheet 2
Moving to the Next Grade

Parents Say

"Every September I feel like we have to start over again. Things that helped my child in school last year have to be worked out all over again."

Teachers Say

"It's a real challenge to get to know each child and their unique needs within the first few weeks of school."

These are common concerns for parents and teachers at the beginning of the school year. However, they are even greater concerns for a student with a brain injury. The educational needs of this student are more complex due to a broad range of learning, behavioral, and physical needs.

Each school district has procedures for passing student information to the educators working at the next grade level. This worksheet is intended to support and supplement them. Since educational programs for the student with a brain injury require close coordination and support in the school environment, this worksheet defines the basic information teachers and other school staff need to start the new school year.

This worksheet can be filled out by either parents or teachers. Often it has been helpful to both because it summarizes the student's needs and identifies the location of assessments, plans, and specialists who have worked with the student.

Student name ________________________________ Date ______________

Age and grade now ____________ Age and grade at time of injury ____________

1. Current educational plan & reports from last school year

List Reports **Dates of Reports**

____

____

____

____

____

____

____

____

____

2. School Work

Work samples

List Samples Attached **Description**

____

____

____

Special books and materials used

List

____

____

____

Adaptive/assistive equipment or interventions

List

____

____

____

Learning style/general strengths and needs

List

____

____

____

____

Behavior affecting learning in class

List

____

____

____

3. Current medical summary

Brief history of injury/illness and medical treatment

____

____

____

____

____

____

Current medications, and side effects

____

____

____

____

____

____

Medical issues at school

List **Methods of response**

____

____

____

____

____

4. Special services provided during most recent school year

Service **Name** **Tel #**

Special education

____

____

Psychology

____

____

Neuropsychology

____

____

Physical Therapy

____

Occupational Therapy

____

Speech/Language Therapy

____

Adaptive Physical Education

____

Counseling/guidance

____

5. List of important contacts

Name **Address** **Phone** **Role**

1. ____

____

2. ____

____

3. ____

____

4. ____

____

5. ____

____

6. ____

____

7. ____

____

8. ____

____

9. ____

____

10. ____

____

Worksheet 3
Moving Between Classes in Middle or High School

Parents say

"I'm worried about my child going into middle school. We've come so far since the injury and worked out lots of support in elementary school. But so much more is expected academically in middle school with a lot more responsibility on the student to get the work done."

"High school is much harder for my son but he's managing. Where he gets into trouble is the little stuff; being on-time, remembering to bring the right books to class, getting anxious about doing something new."

Teachers say

"Most kids this age are disorganized but can get it together when pushed. But the student with a brain injury seems to fall apart under pressure."

Special education coordinators say

"It's tough to communicate every detail of the education plan to all the staff involved. There are over fifteen people working with this student. Sometimes things just don't go smoothly."

Students entering middle school and high school face significant organizational challenges adjusting to many teachers, moving between classes, and managing assignments. These organizational problems can be even more difficult for a student with a brain injury. Learning and remembering how to get around a new school building, what time classes change, what class or activity comes next, or the locker combination, can easily overwhelm this student. Add the physical and mental fatigue that so often accompanies recovery from a brain injury and it is clear that the middle or high school student faces many challenges.

It is critical that a support system be developed to help the student adjust and succeed in middle school or high school. This support system must:

1) be coordinated among all school personnel who supervise the student (teachers, guidance counselors, and aides)

2) provide adequate support and strategies for the student to do school work

3) be understood and accepted by the student.

This worksheet provides a blueprint for planning key issues. This worksheet can be filled out in a meeting with the student, parents, teachers and other staff. A backup plan is included in the worksheet. Situations will come up that can't be anticipated. Steps are listed to help the student "get back on track." The worksheet is signed and circulated to school staff who come in contact with the student.

Student name ______________________ **Date** __________

Age and grade now __________ **Age and grade at time of injury** __________

1. Summary of student's challenges

Issues

1. ____
____

2. ____
____

3. ____
____

4. ____
____

5. ____
____

2. Transition issues to address

Finding way to class (spatial orientation)

Adaptive strategy Person to monitor

____

____

____

Time to move between classes (ample time to get from place to place)

Adaptive strategy Person to monitor

___

___

___

Following schedule (in the right place at the right time)

Adaptive strategy Person to monitor

___

___

___

Time to finish tests/quizzes or other classroom work (adequate time to get work done due to slowed speed of thinking and working)

Adaptive strategy Person to monitor

___

___

___

Managing books/materials (moving, storing, and having books)

Adaptive strategy Person to monitor

___

___

___

Managing homework assignments (coordinate with help at home)

Adaptive strategy Person to monitor

____

____

____

____

____

Learning problems (reading disability, trouble with math or inability to express ideas in writing)

Adaptive strategy Person to monitor

1. ____

____

2. ____

____

3. ____

____

4. ____

____

5. ____

____

3. If these adaptive strategies don't work-what's the backup plan

Procedure to follow   Person responsible

1. ____

____

2. ____

____

3. ____

____

4. ____

____

4. Next meeting to evaluate this plan

Date, time, & location of meeting   Person responsible

____

____

____

5. Acknowledgment and agreement by all participants

Name	Signature	Date
Student	____________________	
Student's parent(s)	____________________	
Home room teacher	____________________	
Guidance counselor	____________________	

Name	Signature	Date
Physical education teacher		
Teacher		
Teacher		
Teacher		
Aide		
Lunch room aide(s)		
Therapists		
Therapists		
Special ed coordinator		
Director of special education		
Special ed teacher		
Case manager		
School nurse		

Conclusion

School is so much more than taking classes and passing or failing. It is the arena where a student develops relationships with peers, faces academic challenges and prepares for life as an adult. So often, whether a student succeeds or fails in school has a powerful impact on that student's self-image and relationships with others. Grades in school are just one of the many yardsticks used to measure the achievements and potential of students. They become a major factor in vocational and academic choices.

There are other achievements that are harder to measure and are not reflected in grades. There is the courage and determination that many students with brain injuries demonstrate as they struggle to adjust to a "new self" while grieving what has been lost. The emotional trauma that accompanies a brain injury is powerful. The close "brush with death" and fear of losing their child is an experience that few parents ever forget. The child's return to school raises many anxieties, fears and concerns for the student and family. It is in school and over time that the long-term consequences of the injury become apparent as the brain matures.

School presents special challenges now. Many students with brain injuries will succeed. Many will have great difficulties. Some will fail. The challenge for educators is to understand the complex and dynamic nature of brain injury, to identify the techniques from their repertoire of educational strategies that are effective for this student, to work with consultants and experts to understand how the student's brain is functioning, and to work with parents as partners rather than adversaries.

Educators have a very special role and challenge as they work with these students. This book has tried to provide an understanding of how the brain works, what happens when it is injured, and what this can mean for the student's ability to learn. The students you teach today are the adults of tomorrow.

References

Blosser J and DePompei R., Second Edition *Pediatric Traumatic Brain Injury: Proactive Intervention*. Clifton Park, NY: Thomson, Delmar Learning, 2003.

Krauss, FJ. Epidemiological features of brain injury in children: Occurence, children at risk, causes and manner of injury, severity, and outcomes. In SH Broman and ME Michel (Eds), *Traumatic Head Injury in Children* (pp 22-39). New York: Oxford University Press, 1995.

Marchese N, Potoczny-Gray, Savage R. *Behavior after Brain Injury: Changes and challenges.* Wake Forest, NC: Lash and Associates Publishing/Training, Inc., 1998.

Moore Sohlberg M, Todis B, Glang A, Lash M. *Brain Injury: Causes and consequences for students.* Wake Forest, NC: Lash and Associates Publishing/Training, Inc., 1999.

Savage R. *An Educator's Guide to the Brain and Brain Injury. In: Educational Dimensions of Acquired Brain Injury.* R Savage and G Wolcott (Eds) Austin, TX: PRO-ED, 1994. Pgs 13-31.

Traumatic Brain Injury Fact Sheet. Washington, DC: National Information Center for Children and Youth with Disabilities, March 2000.

Changes in Self Awareness

Among students with brain injuries

McKay Moore Sohlberg, PhD, Bonnie Todis, PhD, & Ann Glang, PhD ~ 1999

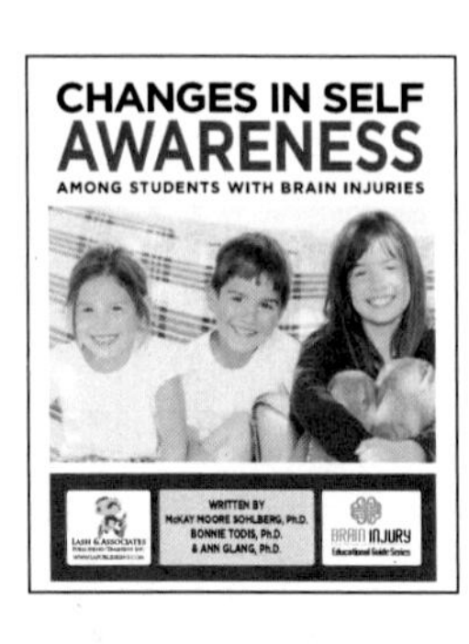

This manual explains five factors that contribute to unawareness after a brain injury. It shows how to work with the student by using awareness activities consistently over time. Awareness exercises show how to:

- build student's awareness of how things are going at school
- understand effects of brain injury on school work and peers
- develop adaptive strategies with teachers.

Item: AWARE 28 pages, 7 x 8½ soft cover

Compensatory Systems

For students with brain injuries

Ann Glang, PhD, McKay Moore Sohlberg, PhD & Bonnie Todis, PhD ~ 1999

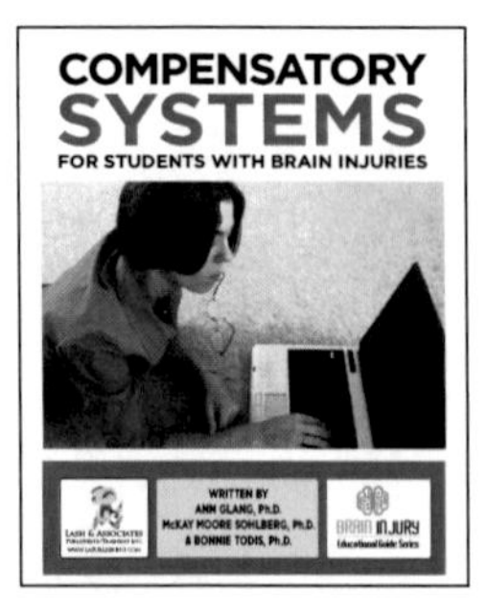

The activities in this manual help educators select a compensatory system, teach students how to use it, and monitor how well the system is working for the student. Includes practical guidelines to help students with brain injuries use compensatory systems successfully. Has forms for selecting a system, monitoring homework, using the system, tracking schedules, and monitoring student notebook.

Item: COMP 40 pages, 7 x 8½ soft cover

Learning and Cognitive Communicative Challenges

Developing educational programs for students with brain injuries

Roberta DePompei, PhD & Janet Tyler, PhD ~ 2004

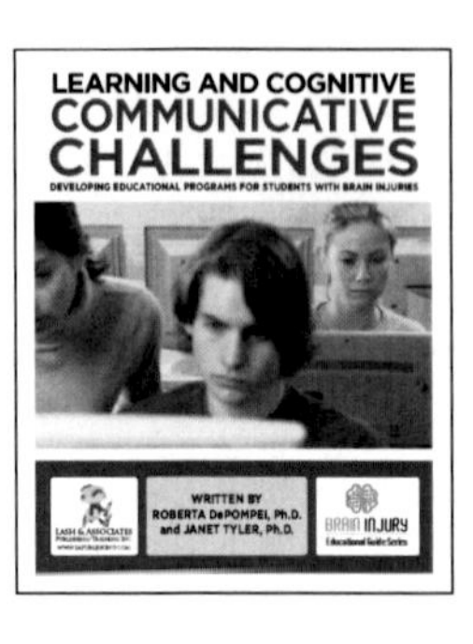

This manual details classroom behaviors cause by changes in attention, processing speed, short-term memory, long-term memory, organization, problem solving, impulsivity, expressive language, receptive language, pragmatic language, and executive functioning. It gives educational strategies for helping the student with language demands of English and Language Arts, Social Studies, Mathematics, and Science.

Item: LCCC 48 pages, 7 x 8½ soft cover

Item: BIEDUSET **Special Price: $50.00**

LASH & ASSOCIATES PUBLISHING/TRAINING INC.
100 BOARDWALK DRIVE, SUITE 150, YOUNGSVILLE, NC 27596
TEL: (919) 556-0300 FAX: (919) 556-0900
WWW.LAPUBLISHING.COM